EXERCISE
and
ARTHRITIS

A Guide to
Pain-Free Movement

Other Books From the People's Medical Society

Alzheimer's and Dementia: Questions You Have. . . Answers You Need

Arthritis: Questions You Have. . . Answers You Need

Blood Pressure: Questions You Have. . . Answers You Need

Hearing Loss: Questions You Have. . . Answers You Need

The Hormone Replacement Handbook

Long-Term Care and Its Alternatives

Medicare Made Easy

Prostate: Questions You Have. . . Answers You Need

Self-Care: Your Family Guide to Symptoms and How to Treat Them

Stroke: Questions You Have. . . Answers You Need

Take This Book to the Hospital With You

What to Do When It Hurts: Self-Diagnosis and Rehabilitation
of Common Aches and Pains

Your Heart: Questions You Have. . . Answers You Need

EXERCISE
and
ARTHRITIS

A Guide to Pain-Free Movement

By
Margaret Hills, S.R.N., and Janet Horwood

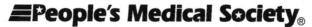
People's Medical Society®

Allentown, Pennsylvania

The People's Medical Society is a nonprofit consumer health organization dedicated to the principles of better, more responsive and less expensive medical care. Organized in 1983, the People's Medical Society puts previously unavailable medical information into the hands of consumers so that they can make informed decisions about their own health care.

Membership in the People's Medical Society is $20 a year and includes a subscription to the *People's Medical Society Newsletter*. For information, write to the People's Medical Society, 462 Walnut Street, Allentown, PA 18102, or call 610-770-1670.

This and other People's Medical publications are available for quantity purchase at discount. Contact the People's Medical Society for details.

Library of Congress Cataloging-in-Publication Data

Hills, Margaret.
    [Curing arthritis exercise book]
    Exercise and arthritis : a guide to pain-free movement / by Margaret Hills and Janet Horwood.
        p.   cm.
    Originally published under the title: Curing arthritis exercise book.
    Includes index.
    ISBN 1–882606–33–7
    1. Arthritis—Exercise therapy. I. Horwood, Janet.
II. Title.
RC933.H52   1997
616.7'22062—dc21   97–17033
                                   CIP

    3 4 5 6 7 8 9 0

First printing, August 1997
Illustrations by Jerry O'Brien

Contents

Introduction

In September 1946, at the age of 21, I started training as a nurse at St. Stephen's Hospital, London. I was fun-loving and carefree; I loved to dance, cycle and swim; and my greatest ambition was to be a good nurse. But early in April 1947, I began to feel unwell. I was taken to the nurses' sick bay, and the doctor diagnosed acute rheumatoid arthritis. It was also discovered that I had a badly enlarged heart, so I was confined to bed and told to have a period of complete rest.

I lay in bed totally helpless for four months, then gradually was allowed to sit out of bed and wash and feed myself. Apart from complete rest, the only treatment I received was aspirin. After five months, I was allowed to leave the hospital to convalesce at home. Before I left, the medical superintendent came to see me. He told me that because I had been very ill and my heart was very badly enlarged, I was never to dance, cycle or swim again. I was not to run uphill or upstairs, and I was not to resume my nursing training because the work was too hard and would tax my heart.

All this was very good advice; indeed, faced with the same set of circumstances, I would probably give the same advice to a patient of mine today—an enlarged heart should not be taken lightly. But I was young and foolish. I decided to ignore all the advice. I resolved to do what I wanted, when I wanted. I resolved to enjoy any time I had left. I danced, cycled and swam at every opportunity. At the end of three months, I was surprised to find that I was still alive.

Becoming a nurse was still my main objective, so I resumed training. Osteoarthritis was beginning to set in, however, and I sometimes suffered great pain. Despite this, I managed to get through my training, and when I had passed my finals, I was given the job of staff nurse in the operating room. Standing for long hours at the operating table proved to be very painful; my back and legs ached, but I carried on. Still, the arthritis got steadily worse. My experience in the hospital had made me realize that the medical profession could not cure arthritis, and the more I suffered, the more fearful I became. The future looked bleak.

Since my original diagnosis, I had researched the possible causes of the disease—including an overabundance of uric acid derived from food and drink. I developed a detoxification program that I now dispense to patients at my clinic. It rid me of all signs of arthritis in just 12 months. That was more than 30 years ago. I have had a wonderful, pain-free life since then, although some stiffness persisted for a very long time. By incorporating a few simple exercises into my routine, I was able to eliminate even this problem. For years, I have had no trouble at all.

The human body is designed for activity—all bodily functions degenerate and atrophy without use—so it is very important that we all exercise properly. But it is especially important for arthritis sufferers to do so. I wish you well in all your efforts to help yourself.

Margaret Hills, S.R.N.

CHAPTER 1

An Arthritis Overview

Nearly 40 million Americans suffer from **arthritis**.† While the disease is generally associated with older people, some forms can strike even the very young. For some people, arthritis is mildly inconvenient. For others, it is debilitating. Arthritis has no cure, and there is no surefire way to prevent it, but there are ways to help relieve the suffering and restore and retain mobility. Exercise is one of the keys. But before we explain exactly how exercise can help you cope with your arthritis, you need to know a little bit about this common disease.

The word *arthritis* literally means "**inflammation** of a **joint**." Inflammation is the body's protective response to an injury or infection. Its symptoms—heat, redness, swelling and pain—are produced by biochemicals that the body's infection-fighting immune cells secrete as they attempt to wall off and destroy bacteria, viruses and other foreign microorganisms. Inflammation can also occur when the body's immune system, for reasons not clearly understood, mistakenly attacks the body's

† Terms printed in boldface can be found in the glossary, beginning on page 110. Only the first mention of the word in the text will be boldfaced.

own tissue. This appears to be the cause of one common form of arthritis—**rheumatoid arthritis**. But inflammation plays only a minor role in the most common form of arthritis—**osteoarthritis**.

Regardless of the amount or cause of inflammation, arthritis affects the body's joints—places where two or more bones meet. Joints are held together by **ligaments**—strong, fibrous bands that connect bone to bone and wrap around joints to keep them stable. To prevent the bones from grinding together, their ends are covered with a tough, rubbery tissue known as **cartilage**. In addition, each joint is encased in a tough, fibrous, fluid-filled **joint capsule**. The cells lining this capsule form the **synovial membrane**. These cells secrete **synovial fluid**, which provides protective lubrication to the joint and helps nourish the cartilage.

TYPES OF ARTHRITIS

There are many forms of arthritis. In fact, more than 100 different conditions are classified as rheumatic diseases—diseases that involve inflammation and degeneration of **connective tissue** and related structures. These diseases can affect the joints and connective tissues in the body, including the muscles, **tendons**, ligaments, heart, lungs, skin and eyes, as well as the protective coverings of some internal organs. They include **gout**, a form of arthritis partial to big toes; **Lyme disease**, a tick-transmitted form of arthritis; **systemic lupus erythematosus**, a chronic inflammation of tissues and organs; **ankylosing spondylitis**, a condition that leads to stiffening of the spine; and **juvenile rheumatoid arthritis**, a form of arthritis that, as the name implies, affects children. The most common forms of arthritis, however, are osteoarthritis and rheumatoid arthritis.

OSTEOARTHRITIS

Osteoarthritis, also called *wear-and-tear arthritis* or *degenerative joint disease*, results from the breakdown of cartilage and other tissues in a joint. Usually caused by joint injuries or aging, it is the most common type of arthritis, typically affecting the hips, knees, feet and spine. Other joints commonly affected include those in the finger, the base of the thumb and the base of the toe, although any joint is vulnerable.

There are several stages of osteoarthritis, all of which can produce pain. In the early stages, the smooth cartilage covering the ends of the bones softens and becomes pitted and frayed. The cartilage loses its elasticity and is easily damaged by overuse or injury. With time, large sections of cartilage may be worn away completely, allowing the bones to rub together. As the cartilage breaks down, the joints may change shape. Eventually, the bone ends may thicken and form bony growths, called **bone spurs**, where the ligaments and joint capsule attach to the bone. Fluid-filled cysts may form in the bone near the joint. And bits of bone or cartilage that have broken loose may drift around in the joint space, causing pain.

In its early stages, osteoarthritis often affects joints only on one side of the body. Later, it may spread to the other side. Symptoms differ from joint to joint and person to person. Some people experience mild aching and soreness in the joints, especially when they move; others develop nagging pain that persists even when they are resting.

RHEUMATOID ARTHRITIS

Rheumatoid arthritis primarily causes inflamed joints, but it can also affect other parts of the body, including connective tissues and the tissues that surround organs. It can develop at any age, but it typically shows up between the ages of 35 and 50. It strikes the joint capsules and inflames the synovial membranes, causing the membranes to thicken, overgrow and become fibrous. These thickened membranes become a harbor for the disease-fighting cells of the immune system, which secrete biochemicals that damage the tissues of the joint. Without treatment, the disease can ultimately erode the cartilage and bone and begin to destroy the joint capsule and ligaments, resulting in joint deformity.

No one knows exactly what causes rheumatoid arthritis. One prevalent theory is that rheumatoid arthritis is an **autoimmune disease**, a disorder in which the body turns against itself and begins destroying its own cells and tissue.

Rheumatoid arthritis can present itself in many ways and can change and evolve over time. About two-thirds of people with the disease first experience fatigue; lack of appetite; general weakness; and mild, intermittent muscle and bone stiffness and pain. Specific symptoms such as early-morning stiffness and painful, hot joints typically appear gradually as several joints, especially those of the hands, wrists, knees and feet, become affected. This usually occurs on both sides of the body. In about one-third of people with rheumatoid arthritis, symptoms may be confined to one or a few joints for months or years, then more and more joints develop symptoms.

The majority of people with rheumatoid arthritis have symptoms that come and go over a course of many years. Some people's symptoms never worsen; others have increasingly severe and prolonged **flare-ups** (periods during which the disease is producing symptoms), then their symptoms settle down, or go into **remission**.

TREATMENT

There is no cure for either rheumatoid arthritis or osteoarthritis. Medical care focuses on relieving pain, reducing inflammation, slowing the progress of the disease, preventing permanent joint damage and keeping joints functional. Treatment may include any of a wide variety of therapies, among them drugs; physical therapy; occupational therapy; psychological counseling; surgery; and lifestyle changes, including exercise.

A properly designed, faithfully performed exercise program can help start you moving and keep you moving. It can improve muscle strength, build stamina and allow joints to move better, with less pain and swelling. And it may give you new energy and optimism. The exercises in this book, performed as recommended by your doctor or **physical therapist**, can help you maintain and increase your **range of motion** and keep your joints and muscles flexible and functional, among other things. We take a closer look at the benefits of exercise in the next two chapters. Let's get started.

CHAPTER 2

Physical Benefits of Exercise

People who make exercise an integral part of their lives seem to have more energy to cope with the demands of daily life. Their hearts, lungs and muscles work efficiently, so they have more stamina. Regular, controlled programs also produce stronger muscles and bones, supple joints, good coordination and better balance. These outcomes help people do more without straining.

People who exercise regularly often look better too. Their complexions are clear and glowing; their hair shines; they have good posture and appear confident. These are all benefits of a good program of enjoyable activity.

Of course, other important lifestyle factors affect our health. Eating a well-balanced diet, which includes plenty of fresh, unprocessed foods and essential vitamins and minerals; enjoying the company of family and friends; using activity and relaxation to relieve any stress; and sleeping better all work together to help make us fully healthy.

If you have arthritis, using regular physical activity to improve your condition may seem out of the question. Even if you have led an active life until recently, you might now be tempted to stop, feeling that limited mobility and pain put you, literally, out of the running. This is not the case. If you have osteoarthritis, regular exercise will *not* wear out your joints and make your condition worse. On the contrary, by moving more, you will increase joint protection by stimulating the production of synovial fluid, which coats the ends of the joints and is absorbed by the spongy cartilage. Like oil, this thick substance lubricates your joints and may help prevent further damage. Lack of synovial fluid reduces protection of the joints and can also contribute to the pain of osteoarthritis.

For all types of arthritis, gently moving the joints and stretching the muscles and tendons are the best ways to relieve strain on painful joints, improve body alignment and help you feel more relaxed and in control of your disease.

You should do a few simple, carefully controlled mobility and stretching movements once or twice each day, even when your joints are swollen and painful. If you suffer from rheumatoid arthritis, take advantage of the times when your arthritis is in remission to put your joints through their full ranges of motion and build muscle strength. This can help prevent stiffening or deformity of the joints. If arthritis affects your back and spine, as in ankylosing spondylitis, keep as mobile as possible.

Rest is also important, particularly during **acute** phases of arthritis; it can help lessen the inflammation. The key is balance. Adjust the amount of rest and exercise according to the stage of your disease and how you feel each day. Too much inactivity makes the condition worse, while too much exercise puts you at risk of exhaustion, injury and more pain. Experts now advise you to exercise as much as you can to increase movement and strength, improve the functioning of the joints and create better all-around physical well-being. But be aware of the temptation to do too much. Learn to listen to your body and know when it is telling you to take things easy.

Ideally, you should do some movements every day. In chapter 6, you will find an easy exercise program that can be carried out each day in just a few minutes. Once you have learned these movements (this will take only a few days), they can easily become part of your daily life—a good habit such as brushing your teeth.

If you already take part in regular physical activity, you may need to adapt what you do. To reduce the risk of damage, replace contact sports such as football and explosive games such as racquetball with activities that put less strain on the joints.

To exercise successfully and safely and to benefit fully from exercise, you need to work on four areas: flexibility; muscle strength and endurance; motor fitness; and stamina. All four contribute to your overall fitness. This is why some apparently athletic people may not be as fully fit as they appear.

FLEXIBILITY

Weight lifters may seem strong, but they are doing little for their circulation and even less for their flexibility—the most important area to work on if you have arthritis of any kind. If your muscles are flexible, you can move easily. Flexibility is reduced when your muscles tighten and shorten because this limits range of motion. In other words, if you do not use it, you lose it. Many adults lose their suppleness through sheer lack of activity, but they manage to get through daily life because there is no specific pain or injury. Nevertheless, they are always at risk of an unexpected strain or sprain because of this stiffness.

If you have arthritis, there may be pain in one or more joints, and you may hesitate to move too much for fear that movement will only increase the pain. The less you move your muscles, however, the stiffer your joints become and the greater the likelihood of increased pain.

If your arthritis is very mild or just in the early stages, keeping supple may well be a simple matter of maintenance. You need to take your joints through their full, natural ranges of motion each day so that you can reach, bend, stretch and turn without strain. The exercises in chapter 6 will show you exactly how to do this safely.

If your arthritis is more severe and disabling, working on your flexibility—using slow, gentle movements—will keep your joints lubricated and prevent further deformation. Some passive mobilizing exercises can be done on bad days—using a pole or hoop to prevent the joint from moving too much. Alternatively, a qualified physical therapist can help you ease your joints into movement.

For those who suffer from ankylosing spondylitis, regular back mobility and flexibility exercises are vital; they will help keep the affected areas as mobile as possible.

Suppleness makes a tremendous difference to everyday life if you have arthritis. It can mean the difference between dependence and independence. Dressing, putting on shoes or stockings, reaching up to a shelf, climbing stairs or getting in and out of a car can be so much easier when your joints are more flexible—and you run far less risk of injury.

MUSCLE STRENGTH
AND ENDURANCE

Muscles and tendons help ligaments support the joints and protect them from injury, so the stronger they are, the more stable your joints will be. If you have strong back, buttock and abdominal muscles, your posture will also improve: You will stand straight with less effort, and your joints will take less of the strain.

Muscle *strength* enables you to move and lift heavy

weights efficiently and safely. Muscle *endurance* gives you the staying power you need to complete simple tasks such as carrying bags of groceries or beating a cake batter without becoming exhausted. Strength and endurance take time to build, but gentle repetitive movements are a safe way to build them.

If you have pain, your natural reaction is to move the affected joint less. Rest is essential from time to time, and it may not be possible to do strengthening exercises on days when arthritis flares up. But even the smallest movement will help prevent muscles and tendons from shortening and weakening. A balance between rest and exercise allows you to retain muscle strength and length without putting the painful joint under too much weight-bearing pressure.

If you are one of the unfortunate few who suffers from **osteoporosis** *and* arthritis, you need to be extra cautious. Because osteoporosis decreases bone density, it also increases the risk of fractures. Essential for you are weight-bearing and resistance exercises such as brisk walking, back strengthening and squeezing tennis balls in your hands. Performed carefully and regularly, these will help maintain bone density and muscular strength at the same time.

MOTOR FITNESS

This part of general fitness is often neglected, but as you age, it becomes more important to work on—particularly if you have arthritis. Pain in the hips, knees or feet naturally affects how you stand (your posture), walk and balance. You may be afraid of tripping or stumbling, especially if the pain makes it hard to lift your feet or bend your knees. Exercises to improve your balance, coordination and reaction time will help you feel a lot more secure.

STAMINA

Stamina is the energy to keep going. The pain and distress of arthritis can be debilitating and tiring. By building up physical stamina, you give yourself an extra boost. Your stamina is largely dependent on a healthy cardiovascular system (the heart and blood vessels) and a healthy respiratory system (the lungs). These systems transport oxygen from the lungs to the muscles and organs; the more efficiently they do this, the more energy you have.

The word **aerobic** is used to describe the system that carries oxygen from the air to the muscles, and aerobic exercise is any form of exercise that helps improve the functioning of this system. Oxygen is transported from the lungs via the bloodstream to the working muscles and organs. Regular exercise results in a heart that pumps efficiently, which means it can respond quickly as soon as extra oxygen is needed. The muscles then use the oxygen, together with the fuel derived from food, to produce a steady amount of energy.

Aerobic exercise is the only way to improve stamina, but you do not have to wear a leotard or jogging suit and risk jarring your joints on a hard floor in order to achieve results! You can improve your cardiovascular and respiratory systems by doing any form of sustained exercise that makes you slightly breathless. Your muscles should also feel a little tired. You will feel this way after walking briskly for a while, cycling (whether outdoors or on an exercise bike), swimming or doing water exercises.

Initially, three to four minutes of continuous (that is, without any breaks) aerobic exercise is sufficient. The length of time can be increased gradually over the weeks. Most experts recommend building up to a 20-

minute session of sustained aerobic exercise three to four times a week as a way of gaining aerobic fitness, and then doing two to three sessions a week to sustain it. As you build up to a full-length session, you can check your progress by using the "talk test." While you do your chosen activity, you should feel that you are working hard—your breathing will be heavier, your heart will beat faster, you will feel warm—but you should be able to hold a normal conversation (count or recite a poem to yourself) without being out of breath. If you are completely breathless, you are doing too much.

Always warm up before exercising and have a cooldown session afterward. This gives the muscles a chance to adapt to the demands made on them. Remembering to breathe deeply and evenly throughout the session also helps.

A bonus of stamina-building exercise is that it burns calories and uses body fat as energy. As long as you do not compensate for extra activity by eating more or drinking alcohol or sugary drinks afterward, you will gradually lose any extra weight that might be straining your arthritic joints.

Another benefit of regular physical activity is that it will make it easier to give up the bad habits that affect your health such as smoking and drinking too much alcohol. You will also sleep better and find you depend less on medications to deal with headaches. All the evidence shows that people who get regular aerobic exercise are at lower risk of heart attack and stroke than people who do not.

CHAPTER 3

Emotional Benefits of Exercise

The trouble with many **chronic** diseases such as arthritis is that you may feel powerless over them. Doctors and other experts tell you that your condition is unlikely to go away. Friends and family urge you to come to terms with the disease and adapt your life accordingly. This may leave you feeling helpless and depressed. Your life seems to be ruled by your arthritis.

You may also feel angry or bitter that you have a chronic illness. You may feel robbed of all sorts of things, including the freedom to do what you want, when you want, without pain. There may be resentment. You may also feel the need to rebel; you may not want to accept your condition and may want to fight it. If you are young, you may feel that you are being cheated when you see others of your own age leading apparently full, active lives. If you are older, you may dislike being told that this is to be expected at your age. Whatever messages you receive, they may be negative and may encourage you to envision a bleak future for yourself.

All these feelings are understandable, and it is good to recognize them rather than ignore them. If you feel very depressed or uncomfortable about your anger and sadness, you may find it helpful to see a counselor and talk things over. Often, those who are trying to be kind and helpful may just reinforce your sense of helplessness and not allow you to be positive. By helping you see things more clearly, a trained counselor may enable you to regain your self-esteem, restore your pride in yourself and what you are achieving, and rebuild your hope for the future.

Exercise can help here: The physical benefits will spill over and benefit your emotional health. The body influences the mind and vice versa. Regular exercise of any kind not only enhances your physical fitness, but it also helps you feel a great deal more positive about yourself and your life. You will begin to feel calmer and more confident in your ability to cope. You will sense that you have gained inner strength. If you follow a safe series of movements and know that each move you make is actually going to help your joints function better and lessen some of the pain, you can boost tremendously your determination not to let the disease get the better of you. The simple decision to exercise is a step away from powerlessness toward independence.

When you are ill, you tend to wait for others to lead the way. You take the drugs prescribed for your arthritis, but you are not really fully involved in the decision to do so: The doctor prescribes the drugs; you take them. However, each time you exercise, you make a positive choice to use your body, to move it and to improve it. You may receive help initially from a physical therapist who will show you the sort of movements you can make. If your arthritis is very severe or well advanced, the physical therapist may be very involved with these movements, sometimes moving the joints for you. This will give you confidence. After this, though, the responsibility to do those movements regularly—maybe two or three times a day—is yours. When you do the exercises, you are making a statement: that you are not prepared to lie down and let your arthritis walk all over you—that you will do what you can to help yourself.

Of course, there will be times when it is hard to think so positively—when the disease flares up and you are in pain. This is when rest and movement are essential. Even at these times, however, you can practice listening to your body, sensing what it needs and making your own decision to rest or to do very simple movements rather than a full routine. Decisions like these take you a step closer to managing your arthritis effectively. You are in control; you are making the decisions.

Most people who exercise regularly talk about the feelings of elation and achievement they have as a result. After a successful exercise session, you may notice that you have extra energy. Each time you achieve just a little more, stretch a bit farther or do a few more repetitions of a movement, your self-esteem will receive a much-needed boost.

PAIN MANAGEMENT

Worry about pain may make you wary of exercise. It may help to think of pain as your training partner—it tells you when you are doing too much and should modify your activities. It's the reason you probably avoid carrying heavy loads, putting pressure on sore joints and working too long without a rest.

Not all pain, of course, is created equal. Sudden, sharp pain is a warning that you have done some damage and need to take immediate action to relieve it. If this happens during exercise, you must stop. The chronic pain that accompanies most forms of arthritis is different: It will sharpen during a flare-up, but the rest of the time, it will simply simmer along. Even during these times, however, there are differences: Some people are blessed with little or no pain for days; others are in pain most of the time.

Of course, pain is a very individual matter—we all have different pain thresholds. What is painful enough to make one person avoid any activity may not limit another person at all. That said, pain is still a warning sign, so you must always take notice of it. There will be times when it will be severe and you will need to rest. At other times, however, exercising gently without straining may actually relieve your pain.

Exercise can help pain in three ways. First, remember that if you keep your joints moving, you encourage synovial fluid to flow in and lubricate them. Second, the rhythmic movements of exercise trigger the release of **endorphins**, the body's pain-relieving hormones. Third, when you exercise, you begin to feel relaxed. Your body naturally tenses up in reaction to discomfort. This tension makes the pain worse, so you tense up more. At the same time, the pain can depress you, and the depression can lead to further tension and, hence, further pain. Exercise can help break this vicious circle of pain, tension and depression in which many people with arthritis become trapped.

If you have arthritis, it is natural to worry that exercise may cause you more pain. This can be a psychological barrier, especially if you have been inactive for some time. You need to rediscover how to trust your body, to know that if you learn to move it in the right way, you will not cause *more* pain, but *less* pain. It may be reassuring to seek help from an expert such as a qualified physical therapist or qualified exercise teacher. He or she can teach you safe and effective movements and show you how to make slight adjustments to your position until you gain maximum benefit from these exercises. If supervised exercise is not possible, the very gentle exercises in chapter 6 will allow you to progress and adapt to moving again in a similar way—very safely, slowly and carefully. Each time you exercise without pain, you will increase your confidence. As this happens, you will feel relaxed and at ease with your body, which will reduce the likelihood of pain.

When you finish exercising, your body may feel tired, especially in the early stages—this is discomfort, not pain. If there is pain in the joints and it lasts for more than two hours after you have been exercising, you are probably doing too much and need either to rest or to exercise less energetically. If there is stiffness in the muscles the following day, you have definitely exercised too hard for your level of fitness.

You could also consider other ways of dealing with your pain so that it does not dominate your life. Relaxation is a very effective way of controlling pain if you remember that tension and anxiety often make you more susceptible to pain. Relaxation techniques, therefore, should become as much a part of your life as the more active exercise movements. They are an ideal way to finish an exercise session, but they can also be done at any time—maybe before you go to sleep or if you wake up in the middle of the night. (See chapter 7 for relaxation routines.)

Some people find that visualization techniques help them cope with pain. You could try something simple, such as thinking of your pain as an enemy trying to conquer your body and imagining an army of pain-relieving cells fighting to overcome it. Or you could use a gentler image of support and comfort that will soothe the pain in the way you might hold and cuddle a child who is hurt or unwell.

STRESS REDUCTION

Stress plays an important role in arthritis. More and more evidence shows that certain types of arthritis such as rheumatoid arthritis are made worse or are even triggered by stress, while the changes produced in the joints that lead to deterioration and osteoarthritis may also be linked to stress. Stress affects a person with arthritis both physically and psychologically. Physically, if you are anxious and worried much of the time, your muscles will be in an almost constant state of tension, making movement of the joints even more difficult. Tension restricts blood flow and the supply of oxygen and nutrients to the body, including the muscles. This causes a buildup of **lactic acid**, which, in turn, causes fatigue and exhaustion.

If your worrying also prevents you from having a restful, uninterrupted night's sleep, it gives your painful joints very little chance to rest and relax. It is natural to worry about arthritis in the early stages—you may not know how it will affect your life, and if you have been healthy until now, being unwell may come as a shock. If you have rheumatoid arthritis, you may not know how long it will last, whether it will go into remission or whether there will be further flare-ups.

Our bodies are well equipped to deal with sudden, short-term stress; they give us the extra energy and strength we need to avoid or escape the danger. When this happens, our blood pressure rises and the heart pumps more blood quickly to the muscles to prepare for action. When the danger is past, everything settles down to normal. But if we have long-term stress, this return to normal does not take place. The result is often exhaustion and fatigue.

Exercise is one good way to relieve stress. The sense of achievement and the boost to our self-esteem that result are very helpful. And as we have seen, the very act of moving around helps us relax. In turn, this will help us sleep better, which should help reduce pain.

SOCIAL INVOLVEMENT

In addition to the regular routines that you will do at home to keep supple and mobile and to strengthen your muscles, consider signing up for an exercise class or some other activity that involves meeting people. You may hesitate at first, especially if you find movement difficult. But most classes these days are noncompetitive. The aim is for all people to do the best they can without straining. No one has anything to prove to anyone else, and the support you receive from others can be very helpful and encouraging.

Illness is often isolating; if you have arthritis, it may mean losing touch with people. Maybe you have had to stop work or go out less because you haven't been well enough. Sharing your exercise with others can create a new social life for you, and you will enjoy that special feeling that comes when a group works together.

Initially, you may feel more comfortable exercising with other people who have arthritis. It is good to share experiences and progress, and you can give each other confidence and a feeling of security. As your mobility increases, however, you may also want to join a more general class, perhaps at your local gym.

In addition to being an excellent way to make lasting friendships, sharing your commitment to exercise with others can encourage you not to give up or miss sessions without a very good reason. There is often an unspoken contract and a shared determination to keep going. If you have never been to an exercise class before, you may benefit from the sense of caring, laughter, fun and friendship that can be found there; it may be something you need.

19

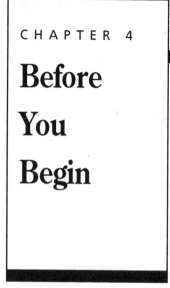

CHAPTER 4

Before
You
Begin

You will need to know how fit and how mobile you are before beginning any exercise program. The following charts can help you prepare for a discussion with your doctor and/or physical therapist.

ASSESS YOUR FITNESS LEVEL

Your fitness level is determined by how active you are. Which of the following is true for you?

Activity Level	Fitness
I exercise aerobically at least three times a week.	Fit
I exercise aerobically at least once a week, or I have an active lifestyle. (I do lots of gardening, brisk continuous walking or going up and down stairs.)	Moderately fit
I am less active than the above.	Unfit

EVALUATE YOUR CONDITION

Next, you should assess how arthritis affects your daily life. Which of the following is true for you?

Condition	Degree of Freedom
My arthritis has no noticeable effect on my ability to do my usual tasks.	Unrestricted
I can do my usual tasks, but my arthritis causes some discomfort and affects my mobility.	Mildly restricted
I find tasks such as dressing and bathing very difficult and need help.	Restricted
I am confined to my bed or a wheelchair.	Severely restricted

CONSULT A HEALTH-CARE PROFESSIONAL

Before starting any exercise routine, please check with your doctor or physical therapist to make sure that you are in good health and that the movements you plan to do are right for you. If you have arthritis of any kind, you must be careful to ensure that the risks of exercise do not outweigh the benefits. This means that the type of exercise, as well as the amount, frequency, intensity and method, *must* be appropriate for your body, fitness level and type and stage of arthritis. Exercise must also be followed with a period of rest to ensure maximum benefits. You may need to adjust what you do every day, but the key is to listen to your body rather than your mind. So avoid exercising a joint when it is particularly painful, especially if you have an inflammatory type of arthritis such as rheumatoid arthritis. In these cases, it is best to rest the joint until the inflammation has subsided.

Remind yourself (and your health-care professional) of what an exercise program for people with arthritis should do:

- It should reduce and relieve any discomfort, stiffness and pain.
- It should prevent further disability, deformity and deterioration.
- It should give you more energy to perform your daily tasks.
- It should increase your self-esteem, confidence and enjoyment of life.

BE AWARE OF THE PITFALLS

No one pretends that it is easy to exercise regularly—all sorts of things come along to make this tricky—but as more and more people have shown, it can be done. It helps to be aware of the pitfalls before you start.

- **Overenthusiasm** is often more of a hindrance than a help. If you are too enthusiastic at the beginning, you may be tempted to push yourself too hard. You may then have pain and be forced to stop. So the rule is to take things slowly and build up gradually; this reduces the chances of injury.
- **Pain** is a natural worry if you have arthritis. You need to understand that if you feel pain while you

are exercising or if you have pain after exercise that lasts longer than two hours, you are overexerting yourself, and your body will not benefit. If you are taking pain-relieving pills for your arthritis, it is very important not to use them to dull any pain so that you can exercise. Remember: Pain is a warning sign. (See chapter 3.) Eventually you will sense the difference between *pain*, a sign that damage is being done, and *discomfort*, a sign that you are doing movements that you haven't done for a long time. This is why we tell you where you should feel the work as your muscles respond. Some exercises may initially be very uncomfortable for you. If this is the case, do not persist. Instead, choose an alternative until you are ready to try again.

- The **plateau** is something most exercisers experience eventually. People often reach a time when they feel that progress has come to a halt. If this happens to you, you may need to make slight adjustments to your routine, say, trying a different series of exercises, finding a new environment or taking up a new activity.

PREPARE YOURSELF

To avoid unnecessary pain or discomfort and to maximize the benefits, you should prepare carefully before exercising. Here are some suggestions:

- Warmth is essential if you have arthritis, so exercise in a warm, comfortable room and wear extra layers if necessary. If you are going to exercise outdoors in the cold, warm up for 20 minutes indoors first.
- Make the room in which you exercise as pleasant as possible.
- Have your equipment (chair, weights, resistance bands and so on) handy.

- Your exercise chair should be a straight-backed chair with a firm seat and no arms. The back should be high enough for you to hold it from behind without stooping. If the seat is at the proper height, your feet will be flat on the ground when you sit on it.
- Have drinking water nearby.
- Have two towels ready—one rolled to use as a cushion under your head, hips or buttocks and the other to mop your brow.
- Take the phone off the hook.
- Wear loose, comfortable clothes.
- Make sure you have a mat or folded blanket if you plan to do any floor exercises.
- Do not exercise immediately after a meal. Allow two hours to digest a light meal and longer if you have eaten meat.

LEARN TO STAY MOTIVATED

Starting to exercise may not be too difficult. You will be full of enthusiasm. Aware of the likely benefits, you probably cannot wait to get started. Although you will feel better almost immediately, it will take time before you notice the physical differences: increased range of motion and strength, less pain and more energy. In the meantime, you will experience these benefits only if you motivate yourself to keep exercising regularly. When you do begin to feel better and stronger, you may be tempted to think you can stop exercising. Be warned—as soon as you give up, the benefits slip away. It may help to remind yourself of these benefits:

- Shoulder movements become larger and easier.
- Arms can be lifted higher with more control.
- Legs become stronger and more stable.
- Breathing during activity is deeper and more even.

- You can do more, for longer, with more energy.
- You will stand taller and straighter as your posture improves.
- Your balance and coordination will improve.
- You will react faster and more skillfully.
- You may be more resistant to infections.
- You will cope better with stress.
- The quality of your sleep will improve.
- You will feel more positive and relaxed.

If you feel you are still losing interest, try one of the following motivators:

- Never say quit—for more than a day!
- Do not let a slip turn into a slide.
- Reward yourself for keeping at it—after one, three, six and 12 months.
- Tell yourself that it's never too late to begin again.
- Remind yourself of the risks of *not* experiencing the benefits of exercise.
- Add up the financial and emotional costs of being dependent on others.
- Imagine the disappointment you will feel if you do not take this opportunity or if you drop out.

Before you start the exercises, here's a final, encouraging thought: When you bought this book, you made a decision to do something more about your arthritis. Now, each time you exercise, you are taking an important step toward being more in control.

CHAPTER 5

The Program Basics

We have divided the exercises in this program into activity segments, or blocks. These can be put together in any combination that suits you (although you should avoid mixing exercises from different blocks). How you do this will depend on how much time you have, what you want to work on that day, your state of health and so on. For example, if you have an hour and are in a good state of health, you could do all of the blocks. Try to alternate between exercises for the upper and lower body—for example, between shoulder and knee exercises. If you are short of time or are in discomfort, you may simply do the warm-up and cool-down blocks. Use the following chart to help guide you.

Activity Block	Duration
Warm-Up	
1 Muscle-Warmers	5 minutes
Warm-Up	
2 Mobilizers	5 minutes
Warm-Up	
3 Stretches	5 minutes
4 Strength-Builders	15 minutes
5 Aerobics	5 minutes *(low level)* 10-15 minutes *(moderate level)* 5 minutes *(moderate to low level)*
Cool-Down	
6 Mobilizers/Stretches	5 minutes

Note: You must always do the warm-up and cool-down blocks.

YOUR EXERCISE ROUTINE

Some people find it helpful to make a timetable and schedule their exercise sessions, including relaxation routines. It often helps to have a definite time that you know you will devote to your exercise. Think of it as you would a business or doctor's appointment—as something that cannot be altered. In order to do this successfully, you could make out a checklist for each day over the course of a week, writing in the exercises in the most appropriate spaces.

Other people prefer to be a little bit more flexible and allot a certain time of day or evening to exercising, being prepared to give or take an hour or so either way. If you put yourself under pressure regarding your exercise routine, you will benefit less since you may spend too much time worrying about getting things absolutely right.

It is probably best to avoid exercising immediately after you get up. This is when you are likely to be stiff. If you are a "morning person" or if your life is such that morning is the only time that you can exercise, you need to get up a little earlier and perhaps have a warm bath and move around to help the blood flow before you start.

If you want to get the most out of your session, you need to be uninterrupted for 15 to 30 minutes. Be firm with the people you live with so that they do not call you to the telephone or the front door. If you are on your own, you will have to try to ignore all interruptions. Your exercises are the most important part of your day; they should have priority.

As you plan your week, the following chart can help you decide when and how often to exercise. It is only a guide, so be considerate and listen to your body. There will be times when you will be unable to reach your planned target, but do not worry. Simply do whichever

Type of Exercise	Sessions per Week	Intensity
Mobility	5-7	Low to moderate
Flexibility	5	Low to moderate
Muscle strength	2-3	Low to moderate
Aerobics	2-4	Low to moderate
Balance, coordination	5	Low to moderate
Posture	7	Not applicable

mobility exercises feel comfortable. If this is too much, concentrate on posture and relaxation instead.

Beginners may be slowed down by several things: remembering what to do, remembering when and how to do it and keeping track of the number of repetitions.

To start with, you may find yourself glancing at the instructions frequently, trying to get the positions right and finding it hard to remember which exercise comes next. If you exercise regularly, though, it is amazing how quickly you can begin to memorize the routines. In the meantime, keep this book where you can refer to it easily.

You do not have to hold positions for precisely the length of time given, but the recommended holding time for all exercises in this book is six seconds. You will soon begin to sense how long this is without looking at your watch or clock.

Counting repetitions can be a nuisance. Most people can manage to count up to five repetitions with little difficulty; after that, ingenuity may be needed. Try speaking out loud, learn to listen to your body and take pride in your technique.

POSTURE POINTERS

THE PELVIC TILT

This essential move places your body weight in correct alignment. It is used for safe and effective standing, lying and sitting and can be done anytime or anywhere.

1. Tilt your pelvis, bringing your lower back under and your hips and pelvis forward.
2. Pull in your abdominal muscles to secure the position.
3. Breathe in as you tighten the abdomen and out as you relax.

STAND OR SIT TALL

Feel the difference in your body, mind and attitude.

STANDING

1. Stand with your feet hip-width apart and toes slightly outward. Be sure your knees are not locked.
2. Do a pelvic tilt.
3. Lift your ribs up and away from your waist and lift your chest.
4. Press your shoulders down and back.
5. Lengthen the back of the neck upward and keep your jaw parallel to the floor.
6. Straighten and lengthen your spine until you are standing tall.
7. Let your arms hang loosely at your sides.

SITTING

1. Sit up straight in your chair with your back away from the chair so that you are sitting tall. Make sure your legs and feet are hip-width apart and your knees are over your ankles, not tucked under the chair.
2. Do a pelvic tilt.
3. Lift your ribs up and away from your waist and lift your chest.
4. Press your shoulders down and back.
5. Lengthen the back of your neck upward and keep your jaw parallel to the floor.
6. Straighten and lengthen your spine.
7. Let your arms hang loosely at your sides.

CHAPTER 6

The Pain-Free Arthritis Exercise Program

Caution: Consult a physician before you begin any exercise program. (See chapter 4.) If you feel any of the following while exercising, stop and seek the advice of your doctor before continuing:

- numbness
- tingling
- dizziness
- nausea
- excessive breathlessness
- pain in the chest, back, neck, face or arms
- sharp pain in the joints

Please read chapters 4 and 5 before you start so that you are well prepared and understand how the program works.

BLOCK 1 (WARM-UP): MUSCLE-WARMERS

CHECKPOINTS

✔ Check that your posture is correct before, and several times during, the exercises. (See "Posture Pointers" in chapter 5.)

✔ Focus on the pelvic tilt and tightening your abdominal muscles.

✔ Make all arm and leg movements in a controlled, rhythmic way.

✔ When you are exercising from a sitting position, never lift both legs at once. Hold your chair seat to support your back, unless you are working your legs and arms in opposite directions.

✔ Breathe easily throughout the warm-up.

✔ Feel your muscles getting warmer and more pliable as you increase your circulation.

CLAP AND SWING

STANDING OR SITTING

1. Pat your thighs six times.
2. Clap your hands together six times at waist height.
3. Rest your hands briefly on your thighs or hips.

Repeat steps 1 to 3 four times.

4. Sway your arms across your body from left to right four times.
5. Rest.

Repeat the entire sequence six times, getting into a rhythm that feels good to you.

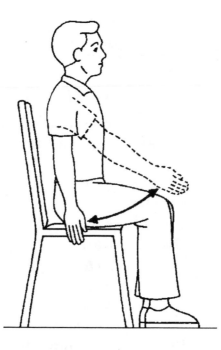

ARM SWING

STANDING OR SITTING

1. Take both your arms forward from the sides of your chair or sides of your thighs to just above the knees or shoulder height in one low swing.

2. Turn your wrists so that your palms face up and lower your arms to the sides of your chair or the sides of your thighs.

Repeat steps 1 and 2 four times.

3. Rest.

Repeat the entire sequence six times, getting into a rhythm.

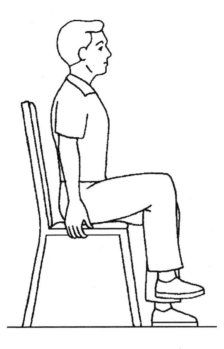

EASY WALKING

STANDING OR SITTING

1. Keeping your feet close together, lift one heel and then the other. Do this 10 times, taking the weight slowly from one foot to the other in a "pedaling" action and keeping the weight distributed evenly between feet. Roll the weight through each foot from the toe to the heel and back. (For chairwork, hold the seat for support.)

2. Rest.

Repeat the entire sequence two times.

ROOM WALKING

STANDING

Progress from easy walking to "traveling" by walking around the room. Start with small, short strides and gradually work up to a moderate pace. Transfer the weight evenly and build up to an enjoyable rhythm. Keep your arms low and move them in the opposite direction of your legs. Do 10 of these longer strides, then return to easy walking.

Repeat the entire sequence six times.

SITTING

Simulate walking by lifting first one knee and then the other. Do this 10 times, then return to easy walking.

Repeat the entire sequence six times.

MARCHING AND BABY ROCKING

STANDING

1. Keeping your movements slow and low, march in place 10 times, swinging your arms in the opposite direction of your legs.
2. Standing with your feet shoulder-width apart and your hips facing forward, sway from side to side 10 times.
3. Bending your elbows, link your fingers together or lay one arm across the other, then sway your arms across your body as though you were rocking a baby to sleep.

Repeat the entire sequence four times.

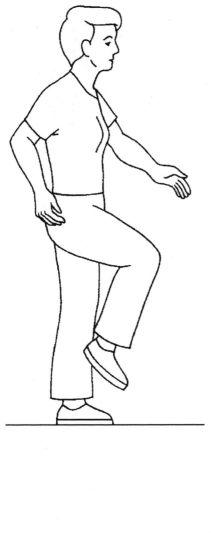

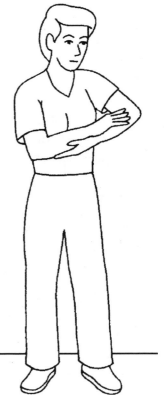

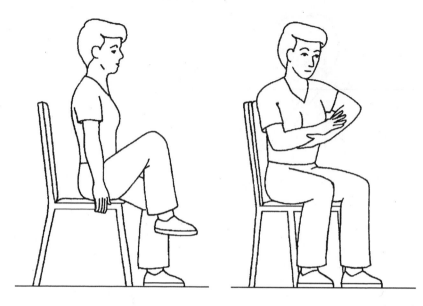

SITTING

1. Keeping your movements slow and low, hold the seat of your chair and move your legs as if you were marching. Do this 10 times.

2. Bending your elbows, link your fingers together or lay one arm across the other, then sway your arms across your body as though you were rocking a baby to sleep.

Repeat the entire sequence four times.

TORVILL AND DEAN

STANDING

1. Pretend you are ice-skating, stepping in a forward direction and transferring your weight from leg to leg. Do this eight times.

2. Sway your arms in the baby-rocking motion described in the previous exercise eight times.

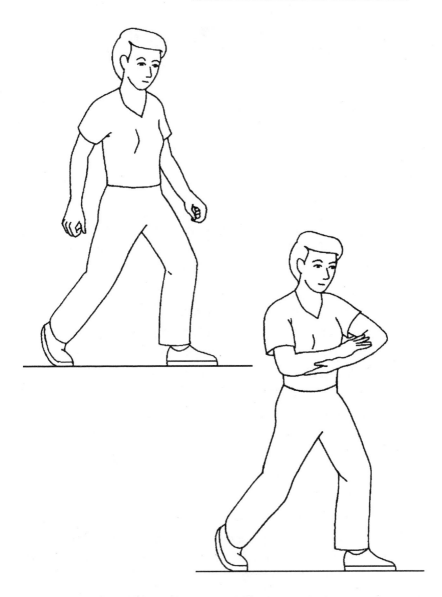

3. Repeat the skating action backward this time, keeping your hips facing forward. Do this eight times.

Repeat the entire sequence four times.

BLOCK 2 (WARM-UP): MOBILIZERS

These exercises, combined with the stretches in block 3, will help you realign your joints correctly, restoring and maintaining their full, natural ranges of motion. They will also improve your posture, allowing you to perform everyday tasks more easily.

CHECKPOINTS

✔ Check with your doctor *before* doing these exercises, particularly if you have had joint surgery or if your arthritis is severe.

✔ Always do muscle-warming exercises first.

✔ Do mobilizing exercises daily if at all possible.

✔ If you cannot do the amount of repetitions suggested, try one or two repetitions.

✔ Always prepare by improving your posture, sitting or standing tall.

✔ Make your movements in a slow and controlled way.

✔ Always work to your full, natural range of motion, but never to the point where exercise is painful.

✔ Breathe easily throughout.

✔ If you experience pain, *stop*. If pain persists or recurs, *stop*. If you have sudden, sharp pain, seek medical advice.

✔ When you do the exercises regularly, notice the differences they make in your daily life, in your ability to bend to pick things up, dress yourself, comb your hair and so on.

SHOULDERS

These two movements feel good and will loosen and lubricate the joints, helping you maintain a good range of motion, release tension in your neck and shoulders and prevent a rounded back.

STANDING OR SITTING
1. Lift your shoulders up lightly, then draw them down, away from the ears. Do this four times.
2. Roll your shoulders forward, upward, backward and down. Hold them in the back-and-down position for a moment, then move the shoulders in a continuous circle, smoothly and slowly.
3. Rest.

Repeat steps 2 and 3 four times.

ANKLES (1)

You will really feel and see a difference if you do these regularly. Your ankle stiffness will decrease, and your ankles will feel looser, especially when you step and stride and go up and down stairs.

STANDING
1. Stand near a wall or the back of your exercise chair; use either to support you.
2. Bend one knee slightly to support your weight safely.
3. With the other foot, put first the heel, then the toe on the floor in a heel-to-toe action.
4. Repeat the up-and-down movement slowly and deliberately, gradually increasing the range of motion of your ankle joint.

Repeat the entire sequence three to five times on each side.

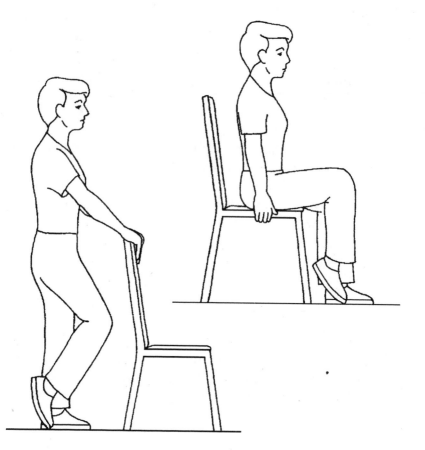

SITTING

1. Sit forward on your exercise chair and support your body by holding the chair seat with both hands.
2. Put your weight on one leg as you put first the heel, then the toe of your other foot on the floor.
3. Repeat the up-and-down movement slowly and deliberately, gradually increasing the range of motion of your ankle joint.

Repeat the entire sequence three to five times on each side.

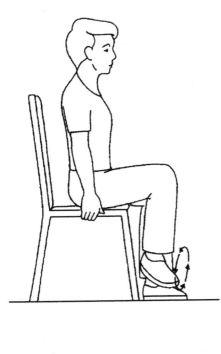
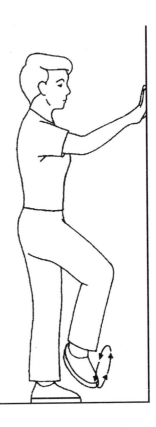

ANKLES (2)

STANDING OR SITTING

1. Stand facing a wall or between two chairs. Use the wall or chairs to support you. (For chairwork, sit forward on your chair and hold on to the seat for support.)
2. Slowly circle your foot—first clockwise, then counterclockwise.
3. Rest.
4. Repeat with your other ankle.

Repeat the entire sequence three times on each side.

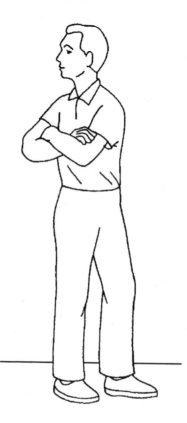

MIDDLE AND UPPER BACK (1)

This exercise is very important for good posture and efficient lung function. Feel your spine become looser, your chest become more open and your back become stronger—and feel the lift in your spirits!

STANDING

1. Stand, legs hip-width apart, with your arms crossed across your chest.
2. Do a pelvic tilt, tightening your abdomen and keeping your hips facing forward.
3. Turn your upper body to the side and turn your head the same direction to look behind you.

4. Repeat, turning to the opposite side.

Repeat the entire sequence four times on each side.

SITTING
1. Sit on your exercise chair with your hips facing forward.
2. Turn your upper body to the right.
3. Rest your right arm across the back of the chair.
4. Place your left arm on your right leg and, keeping your hips facing forward, gently ease your upper body around to look behind you.
5. Move your head around as well so that you are looking over your shoulder.
6. Hold the position for a moment.
7. Repeat, turning to the left side.

Repeat the entire sequence four times on each side.

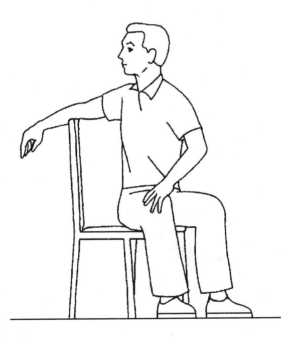

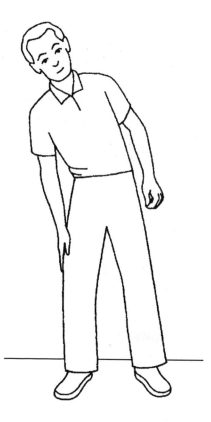

MIDDLE AND UPPER BACK (2)

This will improve your range of motion.

STANDING OR SITTING

1. Slide one hand down your side or thigh, keeping your neck and back in a straight line. Do not lean backward or forward as you do this.
2. Hold the position for two to three seconds, then return to the starting position.
3. Repeat on the opposite side.

Repeat the entire sequence three to five times on each side.

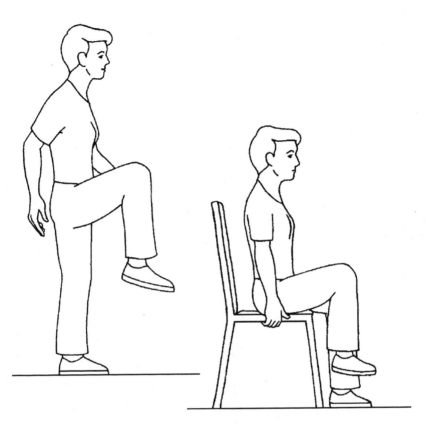

HIPS

Build up the size of the movement you make until you can balance well and can lift your knee as high as is comfortable. Make sure your chest is lifted and your posture is good throughout.

STANDING OR SITTING
1. Slowly lift your right heel straight up so that your knee lifts and bends and your hip flexes.
2. Return your right heel to the floor and lift your left heel.

Repeat the entire sequence 10 times on each side.

KNEES

This exercise loosens the knee joint and is a great one to do every 15 minutes or so if you have to sit or stand for long periods. Build up the size of the movement gradually and perform the exercise slowly and carefully. Concentrate on controlling the leg when you return the foot to the floor.

STANDING

1. Stand near a wall or the back of your exercise chair for support. (Later, you can stand with your hands on your hips for balance.)

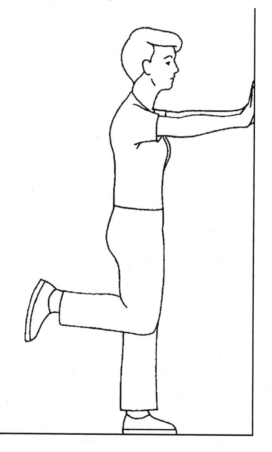

2. Slowly lift your right heel toward your buttocks. Keep your thigh still and do not allow it to swing forward. Avoid arching your back.
3. Lower your right heel.
4. Repeat with the left leg.

Repeat the entire sequence three to five times with each leg.

SITTING
1. Sit on your exercise chair and grasp the seat with both hands.
2. Slowly bend your right knee so that your lower leg is under the chair. Avoid arching your back.
3. Repeat with the left leg.

Repeat the entire sequence three to five times with each leg.

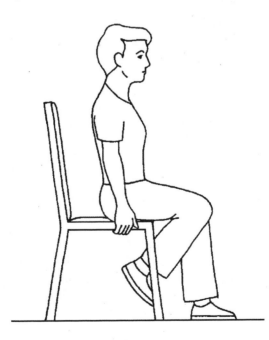

LOWER BACK

This exercise is a wonderful way to care for your back. It loosens and lengthens the lower spine, releases tension and can ease back pain. If you put one hand on your lower back and the other on your abdomen while you do the exercises, you will feel your spine moving.

STANDING OR SITTING
1. Do a pelvic tilt, then bring your rear even farther forward, bringing your hips up toward your nose.
2. Slowly move back to the starting position until you are sitting or standing tall again.

Repeat steps 1 and 2 eight times.

3. Rest.

HIPS AND SPINE

STANDING OR SITTING
1. Standing or sitting tall, tighten your abdominal muscles and lift one hip toward your ribs.
2. Lower it, then repeat on the opposite side.

Repeat the entire sequence several times on each side.

WRISTS (1)

STANDING OR SITTING
1. Tuck your elbows in at your waist and hold your lower arms out in front, at right angles to your elbows, with your palms facing each other.
2. Bring your fingertips toward each other, bending only at the wrists. Keep your hands straight and take your fingertips as far inward as possible.

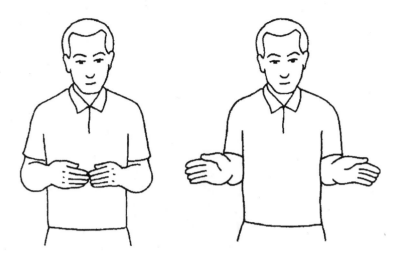

3. Reverse the movement, keeping your arms and wrists in position and bringing the fingertips out as far apart as possible.

Repeat the entire sequence four times.

4. Rest.

WRISTS (2)

Following this exercise, rest by "playing the piano" with your fingers and thumbs.

STANDING OR SITTING

1. Position your arms and hands as in step 1 above.
2. Bring your fingertips toward each other as before. Move your hands in circles from the wrist—up, in, out, down. Do this four times.
3. Rest.
4. Bring your fingertips out as far as possible and

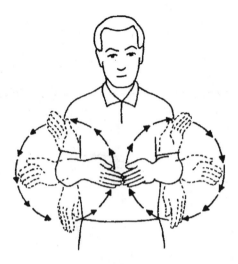

make circles in the opposite direction. Do this four times.

5. Rest.

Repeat the entire sequence.

FINGERS

If you find you have difficulty with your fingers during this exercise, exercise each hand separately, using your free hand to gently assist the fingers of the other hand.

STANDING OR SITTING

1. Adopt the same position you did for the previous exercise, but hold your elbows loosely at waist height.
2. Touch the tip of each finger to the thumb (on the same hand) in turn trying to make round, large "O" shapes in space. Then stretch the fingers out into a wide "V."
3. Rest.

Repeat the entire sequence three to five times.

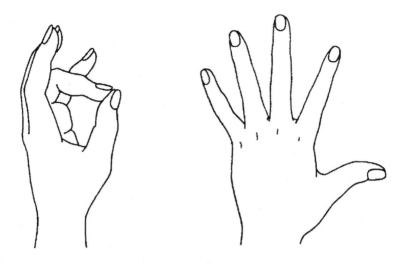

NECK (1)

This exercise and the next one are best done when the body has warmed up a little and any neck tension has been released by previous exercises. Always do these exercises slowly and in a controlled way. Build up the degree of movement in your neck until you are looking as far over your shoulder as possible.

STANDING OR SITTING

1. Look straight ahead and lengthen the back of your neck.

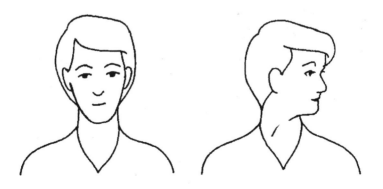

2. Turn your head and look over your shoulder.
3. Hold for two or three seconds and return to the starting position.
4. Lengthen your neck once more.
5. Repeat on the opposite side.

Repeat the entire sequence four times on each side.

NECK (2)

STANDING OR SITTING

1. Looking straight ahead, lengthen your neck and keep your jaw parallel with the floor.
2. Tilt your head toward your shoulder; feel the neck loosening and lengthening on the opposite side.
3. Hold the position for two or three seconds.
4. Lift your head back up to the center again.
5. Repeat on the opposite side.

Repeat the entire sequence four times on each side.

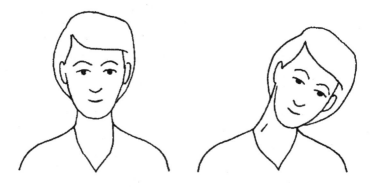

BLOCK 3 (WARM-UP): STRETCHES

HIPS

This is a daily must as it counteracts the negative effects of sitting, helping restore length to shortened muscles and increasing the range of motion in the hips. Ease slowly into and out of this stretch.

STANDING

1. Stand tall, facing the back of your exercise chair or a wall; use either for support during the exercise.

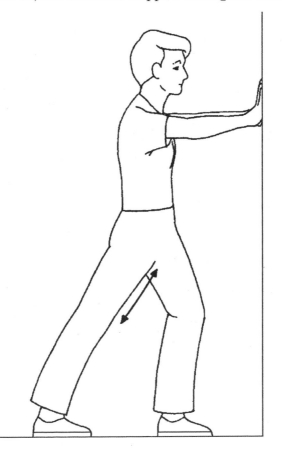

2. With your legs hip-width apart, move one leg back a step.

3. Keeping your feet facing forward, bend your front leg, making sure that the knee does not extend beyond the toe. Keep the back leg straight with the heel on the floor.

4. Tuck your buttocks under and bring your hips forward and up. As you tilt your pelvis, you will feel a strong stretching sensation in the front of the hip of your back leg. Hold for a count of 10.

5. Rest actively by circling your hips gently.

6. Repeat on the opposite side.

Repeat the entire sequence three to five times on each side.

CALVES

This will put a spring in your step and length in your stride!

STANDING

1. Adopt the same position as for the previous exercise.

2. Do a pelvic tilt for good posture and bring your weight forward very slightly. Keep your heels on the floor and feel the stretch in the calf muscle of the back leg.

3. Check the posture of your upper body, think tall and hold for a count of 10.

4. Bring your back leg to the front again and walk in place to loosen your legs.

5. Repeat on the opposite side.

Repeat the entire sequence four times on each side.

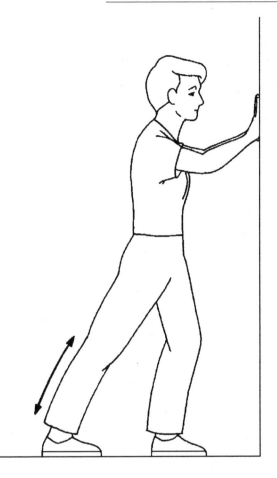

HAMSTRINGS

Another essential daily exercise, this maintains a full range of motion at the hip and makes putting on pants, tying shoelaces and a host of other daily tasks much easier.

SITTING

1. Prepare by improving your posture, sitting tall near the edge of your exercise chair.
2. Straighten one leg in front of you, resting your heel on the floor.

57

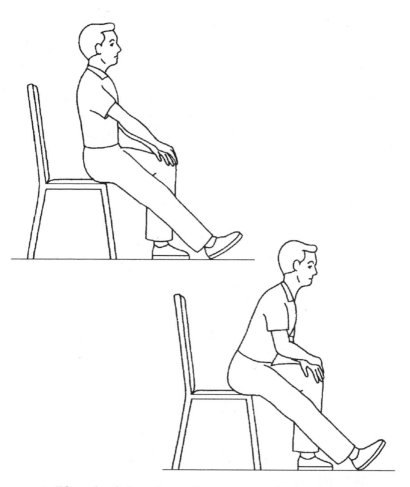

3. Place both hands on the opposite knee to support your back and body weight.
4. Lean your upper body forward and upward until you feel a stretch in the muscles at the back of the thigh (your hamstring) of the outstretched leg. Hold for a count of 10.
5. Rest actively by wriggling your shoulders and hips to release any tension.
6. Repeat on the opposite side.

Repeat the entire sequence four times on each side.

INNER THIGHS

If you have had hip or knee surgery, do not do this exercise.

This makes everyday walking, climbing onto buses and other tasks much easier. It will help you lengthen your stride.

STANDING

1. Stand with your feet apart and your hips facing forward.
2. Bend one leg slightly, making sure that your knee does not go beyond your toes. Keep your other leg straight—but not locked at the knee—and your foot flat on the floor. You will feel a stretch along the inner thigh of your straight leg. If you can't feel the stretch, stand with your feet wider apart.
3. Repeat with the other leg.

Repeat the entire sequence three to five times on each side.

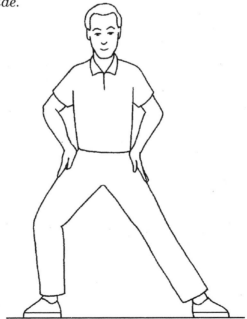

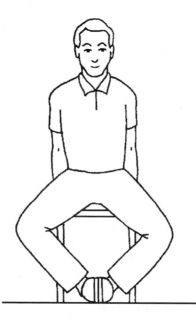

SITTING

1. Prepare by improving your posture, sitting tall either on the floor or on the edge of your exercise chair.

2. Support yourself with your hands either at the sides of the seat of the chair or behind you on the floor.

3. Place the soles of your feet together and allow your knees to fall away from each other toward the floor.

4. Pressing on your hands, gently ease your knees further toward the floor until you feel a stretch along your inner thighs. Hold for a count of 10 and release.

5. Place your hands on your knees and ease gently down for an extra stretch, but do not do this if your arthritis is severe.

Repeat the entire sequence three to five times.

CHEST

This is great for curing rounded shoulders and improving breathing, and it gives you an immediate release of energy. Try to do it five to seven times a week. You should feel the stretch across the chest and arms and the strengthening in your upper back.

SITTING

1. On your exercise chair, sit with your legs hip-width apart.
2. With both hands, reach down and back and grasp the back of the chair.
3. Let your arms lengthen as you lean slowly forward. Keep your ribs lifted, your head up, your jaw parallel to the floor and your shoulders down. Hold for a count of 10.

Repeat the entire sequence three to five times.

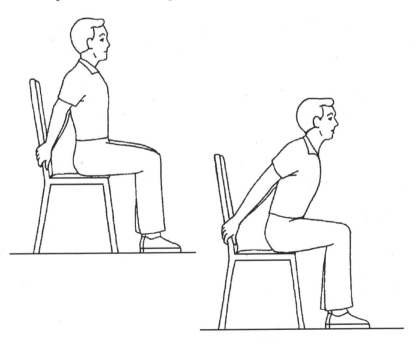

SHOULDERS AND BACK

This will help you continue to zip up and button your clothes, scratch your back and pull clothing on and off with ease. Try to do this five to seven times a week. If you feel discomfort or if your arthritis is severe, take this very easy.

STANDING OR SITTING

1. Lift your right arm straight up toward the ceiling.
2. Bending your right arm at the elbow, bring your hand as far down your back as possible.
3. Take your left arm across your chest and support the raised arm.
4. Ease your bent arm up and back until you feel a stretch along the front of the upper arm. Alternatively, straighten your right arm and bring it across your chest, easing it toward the chest with your left arm.
5. Repeat on the opposite side.

Repeat the entire sequence three to five times on each side.

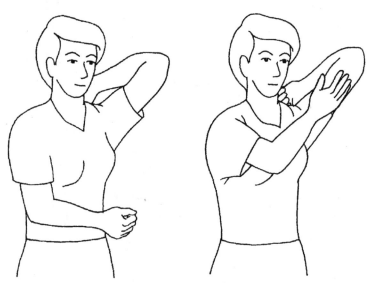

BODY LENGTHENER

This will keep your body tall and improve your posture. Try to do this five to seven times a week.

STANDING OR SITTING

1. As you inhale, extend your right arm toward the ceiling as far as possible, keeping your shoulder down.
2. Breathe out and take your extended arm slightly to the left, over your head, feeling a stretch down your side. Keep your ribs lifted, your back long,

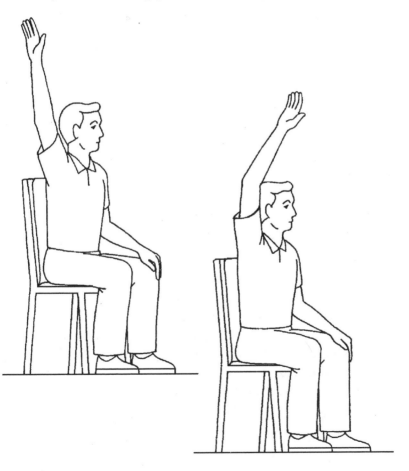

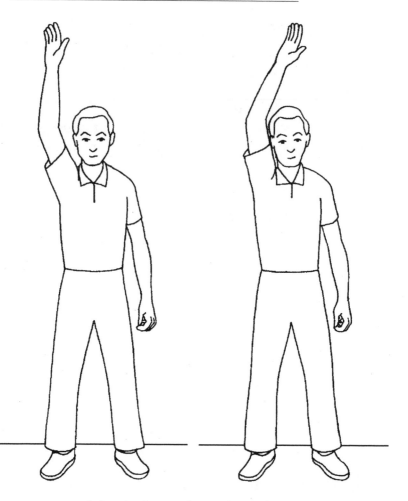

your abdominal muscles tight and your left shoulder down and relaxed. If your arthritis is severe, simply rest the palm of your right hand on your right shoulder and lift your elbow as high as you can or lift your ribs while keeping your hands at your sides.

3. Repeat with the other arm.

Repeat the entire sequence as many times as is comfortable.

WRISTS AND FINGERS

This helps prevent your fingers from curling in. Do the exercise as often as is comfortable.

STANDING OR SITTING
1. Spread the fingers of one hand out wide and flat, as though spanning piano keys. Hold for a count of six.
2. Rest.
3. Spread the fingers out wide as before and place the palm of your other hand under them, avoiding the fingertips. Press lightly on your outspread hand and hold for a count of 10.

Repeat the entire sequence two times with each hand.

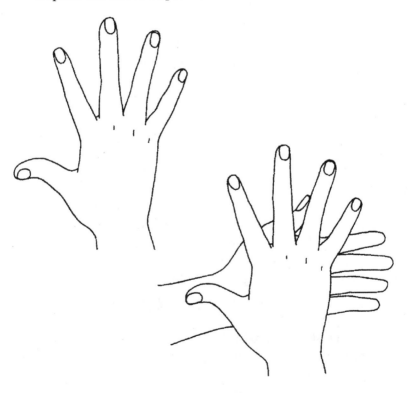

BLOCK 4: STRENGTH-BUILDERS

These exercises are important because they strengthen the bones and the muscles that support the joints, improve posture and body functioning and help you do everyday tasks more easily. Try to do two or three nonconsecutive days of strengthening exercises a week. On difficult days, do just one repetition.

EQUIPMENT

You will need a few pieces of equipment, but they do not have to be expensive. Have your equipment ready before you begin each exercise session.

Resistance bands. Support tights tied together at the ends are an inexpensive substitute. (You can use old bicycle inner tubes when you are stronger.) Always tie bands with a bow rather than a knot because bows are easier to untie.

Weights. You can use canned goods, bags of rice, sand, flour or similar items as weights. Manufactured weights come in various colors and sizes. You should begin with 1-pound weights and work up to larger ones as you become fitter, but do not exceed 5-pound weights.

CHECKPOINTS

✔ **Prepare for each exercise by improving your posture, sitting or standing tall.**

✔ **When holding a position, do not hold your breath—keep breathing easily throughout.**

✔ **Never hold a position for longer than a count of six as your blood pressure may begin to rise a little.**

✔ **Start slowly and progress gradually. Do the exercises for about a month before progressing to the next stage.**

SIDES OF SHOULDERS

You will feel the muscle working at the top and side of your shoulder. Keep a good pelvic tilt and tighten abdominal muscles throughout.

STANDING OR SITTING
1. Hold a weight in one hand or attach one hand to your opposite foot with a resistance band.
2. Keeping your elbow slightly bent, raise your arm out to the side to shoulder level.
3. Slowly lower your arm back to your side.

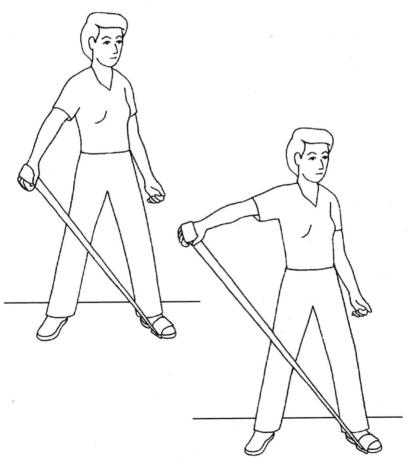

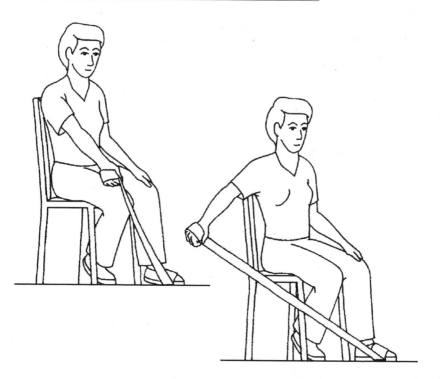

Repeat steps 2 and 3 until your arm begins to tire.

4. Rest.
5. Repeat on the opposite side.
6. Rest actively by shrugging your shoulders to loosen any tightness.

Repeat the entire sequence two times on each side.

SHOULDERS AND ARMS

This exercise helps straighten rounded shoulders and lessen strain on the upper spine. It also opens the chest and increases the range of motion of the shoulders. You will feel the muscles working at the top and back of your shoulders and upper back.

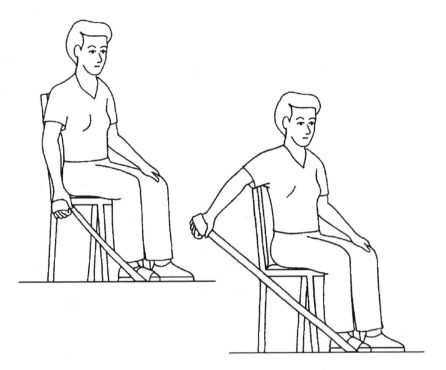

STANDING OR SITTING

1. Hold a weight in your right hand or attach your right hand to your right foot with a resistance band.
2. Keeping your elbow slightly bent at your side, take your whole arm up and to the back.
3. Hold your arm at the farthest point for one second, then slowly lower your arm to the starting position at your side.
4. Rest for two seconds.

Repeat steps 1 to 3 until you feel tired.

5. Repeat on the opposite side.
6. Rest actively by shrugging your shoulders to loosen any tightness.

BACKS OF ARMS

When toned, the much-neglected muscles on the backs of your arms will help you safely lift heavier objects, especially from high cupboards. This exercise will help these muscles (triceps) support the shoulder joint and strengthen the bones in the shoulder and arm. The exercise may also take away that loose, wobbly look from the underarm!

STANDING

1. Face a wall with your arms out in front of you at shoulder height and your palms on the wall, directly in front of your shoulders, with your fingers facing upward.
2. Check that your posture is good. Do a pelvic tilt, keeping your abdominal muscles pulled in to avoid arching your back, then slowly bend your elbows to lower your body toward the wall.
3. Push yourself slowly back to the starting position.

Repeat steps 2 and 3 six times, breathing easily throughout.

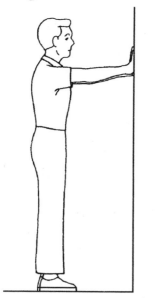 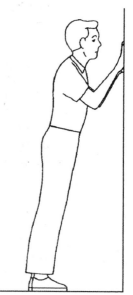

4. Rest actively by shrugging your shoulders and shaking your wrists.

Repeat the entire sequence.

As this becomes easier, increase your fitness by placing your palms farther apart. After several months, take another step away from the wall.

SITTING
1. Holding a weight in each hand, move your arms and shoulders down and back as far as possible.
2. Bend your arms so that your lower arms are at right angles to your upper arms. Your palms should face upward.
3. Keeping your upper arms close to your side, straighten your arms. Hold for a second, then return to the starting position.

Repeat steps 2 and 3 six times.

4. Rest actively by shrugging and rolling your shoulders and shaking your wrists.

Repeat the entire sequence three times.

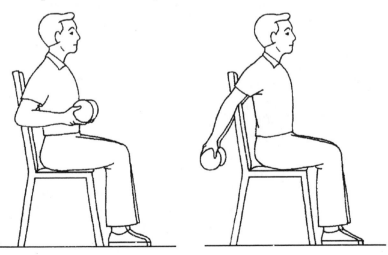

WRISTS

This is wonderful for weak wrists. It strengthens them and will make unscrewing jars and bottles much easier!

STANDING OR SITTING

1. Holding a towel or rubber mat between your hands, make squeezing and wringing movements, as if you were trying to get rid of as much water as possible. Do this first in one direction, then the other until your wrists begin to tire.
2. Rest actively by shaking your wrists and rolling your neck gently from side to side. (Never roll your neck to the back.)

Repeat the entire sequence four times.

SITTING

1. Rest your arms on your thighs.
2. Using a tennis ball or a small towel rolled into a ball, squeeze and release with one hand until you tire.
3. Repeat with the other hand.

Repeat the entire sequence four times with each hand.

CHEST

Use either weights or a resistance band for this exercise. Take care to keep your abdominal muscles tight, your back long and your knees soft (slightly bent) as you do the exercise. Feel the muscles working in your chest.

STANDING OR SITTING

1. Hold the weights in your hands, palms down, or place the band around your upper back with the ends in your hands, pulling it taut.

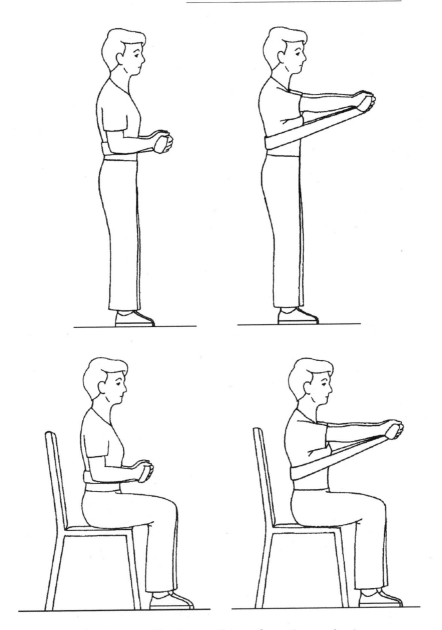

2. Bend your elbows, tucking them in against your
   waist, and hold your lower arms at right angles to
   your body.

3. Press your arms out in front until they are parallel with the floor, just below shoulder height. Hold for a second.
4. Slowly bend your elbows until you return to the right angle and, finally, lower them slightly.
5. Rest actively by shrugging and wriggling your shoulders to release any tension.

Repeat the entire sequence two times.

BACK AND REAR SHOULDERS

This is one of the most effective exercises for straightening rounded shoulders. It also helps reduce pressure on the joints and greatly increases the range of motion and strength of the muscles in both the shoulders and back. If the movements feel uncomfortable, do the exercise without weights or a band.

STANDING OR SITTING
1. Hold a weight in each hand, palms down, or a resistance band in front of your chest.

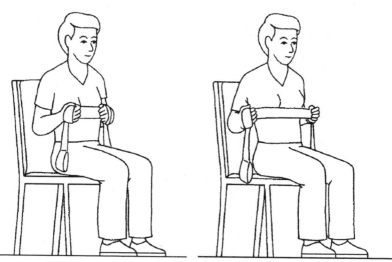

2. Draw your shoulders and elbows back toward your spine, pulling your shoulder blades together, and hold for a count of three. Feel the muscles at the back of your shoulders and in your upper back working.
3. Return to the starting position.

Repeat steps 1 to 3 six times.

4. Rest actively by shrugging your shoulders to release any tension.

KNEES AND FRONT OF THIGHS

This exercise stabilizes the knee joint by working the quadriceps, the thigh muscle that helps the knee track correctly. Indeed, many knee problems are caused by poor tone in this muscle. Do this and the next exercise regularly for the maximum beneficial effect.

SITTING
1. Sit with your legs together and loop a resistance band once around the instep of your right foot,

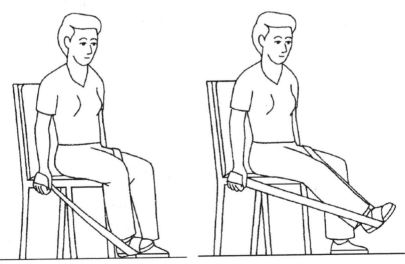

pulling it taut. Hold the ends of the band securely under your hands, resting your palms on the sides of the chair seat.

2. Extend your leg in front of you against the resistance exerted by the band. Move smoothly and take care to avoid locking the knee. Hold the position for two seconds. Feel the muscle in the front of your thigh working.

3. Return to your starting position.

Repeat the entire sequence until your muscles begin to tire.

LEGS AND BUTTOCKS

This exercise helps you maintain your independence and mobility.

STANDING
1. Sitting tall at the front of your exercise chair, tighten your abdominal muscles.
2. Prepare to move after a slow count of three.
3. Lean forward to shift the weight over your hips, then stand up, letting your thighs do all the work. Keep your head up throughout.
4. Stand tall.
5. Steady yourself, then reverse the movement by keeping your body upright, bending your knees and lowering yourself slowly and carefully back onto the chair. Feel the muscles in the front and back of your thighs and buttocks working.
6. To start with, you may wish to place your hands on your thighs (not on the chair) to help you get up and sit down, but gradually lessen the pressure until you are relying only on leg power.

Repeat the entire sequence until your muscles begin to tire.

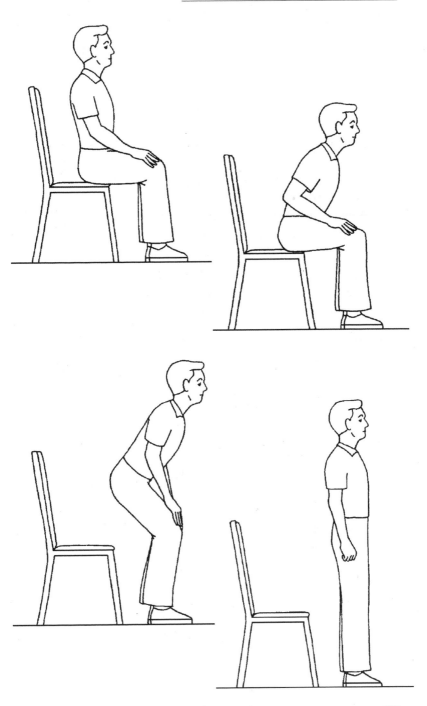

CALVES

If this exercise is too much for you, do extra ankle-mobilizer and leg-strengthener exercises (see pages 41-43 and 76-77) until your legs and feet are stronger.

STANDING

1. Stand facing the back of your exercise chair or a wall and shift your body weight slightly forward, lifting your heels and rising on the balls of your feet as far as you can.
2. Lower yourself back to your starting position with control, using the chair or wall for support if necessary. Make sure you shift the weight gradually right through the feet, from heel to toe and back again. Keep your weight mainly on your big and second toes and avoid placing it on your little toes.

Repeat the entire sequence until your calves begin to tire, then walk in place to release the built-up tension in these muscles.

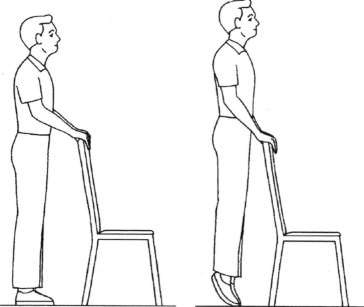

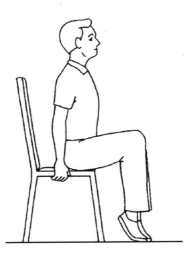

SITTING

1. Sit forward on the edge of your chair.
2. Reach behind you and grasp the sides of the chair seat for support.
3. With a controlled motion, lift your heels.
4. Lower your heels.

Repeat the entire sequence until your calves begin to tire.

HIPS (1)

This exercise helps you increase the range of motion of your hips and strengthens your buttock muscles so that you can take unnecessary weight and strain off the hip joint.

STANDING

1. Connect your ankles to each other with a resistance band, tie small bags of rice or sand around your ankles or attach ankle weights.
2. Stand with your feet about 18 inches away from a wall for support, with your arms out in front of you at shoulder height and your palms resting on

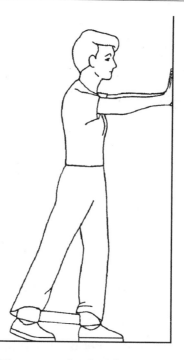

the wall. (You may also hold on to two sturdy chairs to support and balance yourself.)

3. Make sure your weight is evenly distributed between both legs; check that your posture is good and your abdominal muscles are tight; and keep your knees slightly bent throughout, then prepare to move after a slow count of three.

4. Keeping one foot in place, try to press the other leg backward along the floor as far as possible. (You may lift the leg a little as you do this, but think of going back rather than up.) The movement should be small, but controlled.

5. Hold your position at the farthest point for a count of six, then return to your starting position.

6. Repeat with your other leg.

Repeat the entire sequence until your muscles begin to tire.

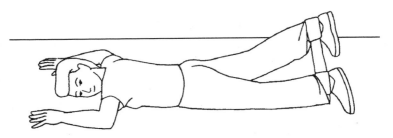

ALTERNATIVE

Lie facedown on the floor, with or without the band or weights, and make the same movement. Never lift both legs at the same time.

HIPS (2)

Make the movement in a slow, controlled way, feeling the muscles in the outside of the hip and buttock working.

STANDING

1. Position yourself as at the start of the previous exercise.

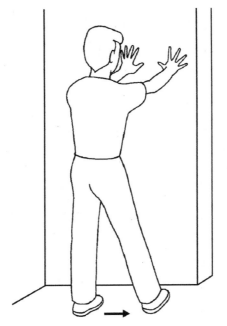

2. Prepare by improving your posture. Place your feet and legs two inches apart, then tighten your abdominal muscles and prepare to move after a count of three.

3. Using the wall or chair for support, press one leg sideways along the floor as far as you can without lifting your hip. Keep your knees and toes facing forward, with your ankle leading the sideways movement. Your leg and foot may lift a little, but concentrate on going along the floor *sideways* rather than up.

4. Return to the starting position, then repeat with your other leg.

Repeat the entire sequence until your muscles begin to tire.

SITTING

1. Sit with your back supported against a wall and pillow for comfort.

2. Beginning with your feet two inches apart, slowly

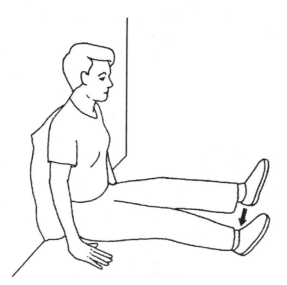

spread them until they are 10 inches apart. Keep them in contact with the floor throughout and be sure your abdomen stays tight to support the back.

Repeat the entire sequence until your muscles begin to tire.

ABDOMEN AND UPPER BODY (1)

This exercise and the one that follows are vital for good posture and a strong back. They will also make your abdomen flatter. You can do them anytime, anywhere, and soon feel and see the difference!

1. Lie on your back with your legs hip-width apart, your knees bent and your feet flat on the floor. Rest your palms on the fronts of your thighs.
2. Check your posture, ensuring that your back is long and pressed into the floor and that your abdominal muscles are tightened.
3. Lift your shoulders off the floor as you slide your fingers up toward your knees, making sure your

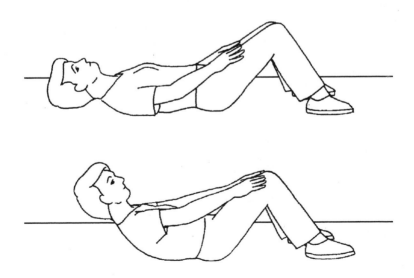

neck is long so that there is a good space between your chin and chest. Breathe out as you come up and pull your abdomen in; breathe in as you lower. Follow the breathing instructions and do not come up too far, too fast. If your neck is uncomfortable, support it with one hand, but don't lock your hands behind your head to pull yourself up—you will risk injury.

4. Lower yourself slowly and with control back to the floor.

Repeat steps 3 and 4 five times.

5. Rest.

Repeat the entire sequence three times.

ABDOMEN AND UPPER BODY (2)

STANDING OR SITTING

1. Bend your knees, making sure not to bring them over your toes.
2. Do a pelvic tilt, check your posture and tighten your abdominal muscles.
3. Pull your abdomen in hard toward your spine while allowing it to curve under a little. Keep your chest lifted and relaxed. Hold for a count of six.
4. Release.

Repeat steps 1 to 4 ten times.

5. Rest.

Repeat the entire sequence three times.

BLOCK 5: AEROBICS

These exercises are vital for a healthy heart and lungs. They are like the exercises from block 1, but the movements are bigger, more vigorous and more energetic. They are aerobic, which means you will require more oxygen to perform them.

CHECKPOINTS

✔ **Discuss your intended program with your doctor or physical therapist before you start it.**

✔ **Always do a warm-up session before and a cool-down session after these exercises.**

✔ **Build up and ease down gradually, making a quarter of your session low intensity, half of your session moderate to hard intensity and a quarter of your session moderate to low intensity.**

✔ **Do movements that use your legs and arms rhythmically.**

✔ **Never stop suddenly; always ease down, making your movements gradually smaller until you are walking, then gradually slowing to a stop.**

✔ **Wherever possible, exercise on carpet, grass or some other springy surface.**

✔ **Wear loose, comfortable clothes and suitable footwear, preferably with shock-absorbing soles. Never work in just socks.**

✔ **Have water nearby to drink during and after the exercises.**

CLAP AND SWING

1. Make big arm movements, clapping at waist level, chest level, head level and overhead.
2. Make your whole body sway as you swing your arms across your body, from right to left, at waist height, shoulder height and, finally, head height. Perform all sways and swings with control.

SWING TURN

1. Sitting on your exercise chair, swing your arms forward, building up to bigger and bigger movements, from hip-high swings to shoulder-to-head-high swings, even swinging yourself up off the chair and onto your feet if possible.
2. Sway as in the previous exercise.
3. Circle your arms over your head and travel around to the right.
4. Repeat the swaying movements, then circle your arms over your head and travel around to the left.

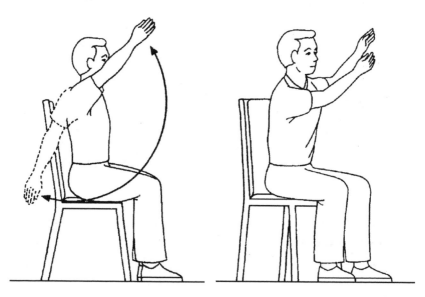

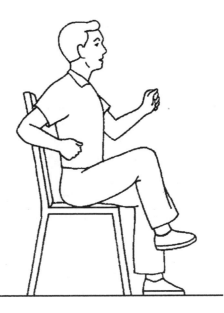

EASY WALKING

Use this exercise to get your breath back.

1. Sit or stand tall with your feet close together.
2. Lift one heel, then the other, taking the weight slowly from one foot to the other in a "pedaling" movement and distributing the weight evenly between your feet as you do so.
3. Build up to a rapid foot-pedaling speed and pump your arms forward and back in the opposite direction of your legs.

ROOM WALKING

1. Walk around the room, transferring your weight evenly as in the previous exercise.
2. Build up to a vigorous walking rhythm, lengthening your stride and swinging your arms.
3. Vary the speed in bursts to get the circulation going.

MARCHING AND BABY ROCKING

1. Stand tall and march in place, swinging your arms in the opposite direction of your legs. Build up to a moderately vigorous marching action.
2. Do this briefly in place, then travel in a circle, lifting your knees as you march.
3. Every now and then, march your feet out until they are shoulder-width apart, then march in this position.
4. Stand with your feet shoulder-width apart and sway from side to side, swinging your arms as if

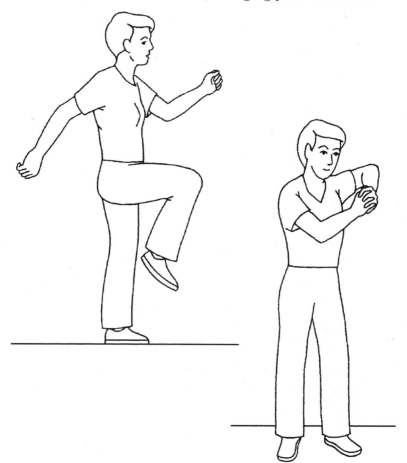

you were rocking a baby to sleep. Swing quite a long way with control from side to side until your muscles feel warm.

5. Finish with some more marching in a circle, lifting your knees and swinging your arms as before.

TORVILL AND DEAN

Pretend you are ice-skating, bending your knees, stepping forward and transferring your weight from one leg to the other while swinging your arms across your body. Bend more deeply and push more forcefully with your legs than you did during the warm-up session.

Remember to bring these actions down gradually until you are back to an easy stage before going on to block 6.

For suggestions of aerobic activities that are enjoyable and beneficial to your health and that you can do in addition to the exercises given in this chapter, see chapter 8.

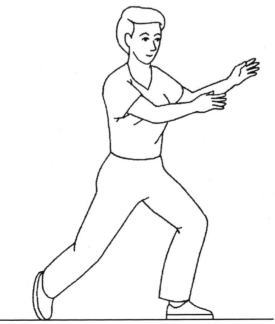

BLOCK 6 (COOL-DOWN):

MOBILIZERS AND STRETCHES

Choose some mobilizer exercises from block 2 and stretches from block 3 and do these gently for five minutes. Then engage in a relaxation activity (see next chapter) to complete your workout.

CHAPTER 7

Rest
and
Relaxation

Learning how to relax is an important part of managing your life—with or without arthritis, but especially with. As mentioned earlier, stress makes pain harder to cope with, so you can make the pain easier to manage if you can find effective ways to relax your body and your mind.

Research has shown that several very useful things happen to your body when you relax totally. Your pulse and breathing rates slow down, you use less oxygen, and blood pressure drops to lower levels. The brain is also affected. When your brain is busy and active, beta waves are recorded. When you are truly relaxed, however, alpha waves and sometimes, in periods of very deep relaxation, very slow theta waves interplay. Alpha and theta waves refresh and restore your body and mind.

You can practice relaxation techniques at any time, but the best times are first thing in the morning (before breakfast) since this prepares you for the day, and at bedtime (at least two hours after your evening meal) since this improves the quality of your sleep. But you can also relax very effectively after your exercise sessions or at any other time during the day. When you get really good, you can use the techniques on a "catnap" basis, whenever you need extra energy.

No equipment is needed, but most people find that they relax best in a peaceful environment where there is very little noise or light and few other people to distract them. Unplugging the telephone is a good idea. If this is not possible, take the phone off the hook, turn off the ringer or cover the phone with cushions to muffle the noise. Some people find that they can ignore outside noises and can even relax effectively on a noisy commuter train or in the office during the lunch hour with phones ringing, while others are disturbed by the slightest sound. You will know best what you can cope with, so arrange things accordingly. You will also improve with practice and find that it is well worth working at.

You need to be comfortable. You do not have to lie on the floor to relax; you can sit cross-legged or on your bed, your favorite armchair, even a straight-backed chair— anywhere as long as you can feel at ease. Ideally, you should relax for 10 to 20 minutes, but even two minutes is better than nothing! You may also like to choose an object to concentrate on, such as a lit candle, a flower or a simple diagram or pattern. Position the item in front of you. Alternatively, you can use a thought, a word, a prayer, the sound of birds singing, a tape of waves breaking on the seashore, a clock ticking, your own breathing or any other rhythmic sound that appeals to you.

Before you start your relaxation session, make sure that you are physically at ease. This means that you should do all the things that might later distract you such as going to the bathroom, blowing your nose so that you can breathe easily, changing into loose-fitting clothes, warming the room or letting in some fresh air, and having a drink.

When you are ready, start by breathing easily—in through the nose, out through the mouth. Maintain this type of even, rhythmic, gentle breathing throughout the session. You may find it helpful to count your breaths from one to 10 each time you breathe out. This is particularly useful if you have a lot of distracting thoughts. Alternatively, you can fill your mind with a visualization of your breath, following its course through your nose, down the larynx, into your lungs and out again.

Next, work toward having no thoughts in your head other than those about your meditation object. Of course, it takes time for you to be able to do this; at first, thoughts of all kinds will crowd into this conveniently empty space. Do not fight them—let them come and go and return your concentration to your chosen object.

Some people find it easier to achieve a state of full relaxation if they do a guided series of movements. For example, you can start with your hands, then move on to your arms, shoulders, upper body, lower body, thighs, knees, feet, neck and face, tensing each part, then relaxing it so that you can feel the difference.

To start with, you will probably find it easiest to try to relax for about three to four minutes, but with practice, you will find you can extend this to 10 minutes and beyond. Do not worry if you fall asleep—you obviously need the rest—but continue the relaxation session when you wake. It is important to allow time at the end of the session to begin moving again. Gradually get your body up and going with some gentle mobilizing and allow the benefits you have received to drift on into the next thing you are doing. You will find that your movements will be slower and you will feel more at peace.

CHAPTER 8

Other Forms of Exercise You Can Do

The exercise routines given in chapter 6, if done regularly and followed by rest, will help you attain better health. Hopefully, you will find that exercise is quite irresistible and will want to do other activities as well. These will further improve your overall fitness and, equally important, be really enjoyable.

Some activities are not recommended if you have arthritis, simply because they can exacerbate your joint problems. Anything that involves sudden, violent movements and is impact based—racquetball, tennis or intense jogging, for example—can do more damage to your joints. You should also avoid exercises that involve kneeling or jumping.

When you have chosen one or more activities, try not to be too enthusiastic when you start. It's easy to overdo it because there is always a temptation to do that bit more, to go that little bit beyond your capacity, especially if you enjoy what you are doing or are determined to improve. Remember: Your body may have become very unfit while you have been coping with arthritis. Even people *without* joint problems run the risk of injury if they overdo things; people with arthritis are even more vulnerable.

Do not let this deter you from trying something new. There are many activities you can enjoy that will supplement the exercises in this book. Some activities such as swimming or walking are an extension of these exercises, while others such as tai chi offer something quite different. Some are more active and demanding, while others allow you to extend your range through gentle movements. The choice is yours; just bear in mind the above safety guidelines.

Many people take up new activities, but large numbers drop them shortly afterward. Since you have decided to make exercise an essential part of your life, you need to ask yourself a few questions before starting an activity if you are to avoid joining the dropouts!

- *How accessible is it? Can you take part as often and as easily as you intend?* The easier it is to get to and the more convenient the timing, the more likely you are to keep doing it.
- *Does it fit into your life and the time you have available?* If you lead a busy life and choose an activity that takes a lot of time either to get to or participate in, you may find you cannot continue to fit it into your schedule.
- *Is it expensive?* Before you invest in special equipment or lessons, you need to feel committed.
- *Is it dependent on the weather?* If you choose something that you can do only on dry days, be prepared to find alternatives when the weather is against you.
- *Will you meet other people?* This is important for people who like to exercise with others for encouragement and socialization.

The secret of success is to choose something that you enjoy doing—something that leaves you feeling fulfilled, refreshed and happy, rather than exhausted and frustrated. You do not have to commit yourself to just one activity—if you have the time or the inclination, you can participate in two or three. For instance, you might choose to go swimming one day, walk two others and take a tai chi class on the weekend. After several weeks, you may find that you prefer and want to concentrate on a single activity, or you may be happy to continue with a variety of activities.

What you choose will depend on what is available in your area and how advanced your arthritis is. The following pages will guide you through some of the likely options to help you make your own choices. No matter which activity you choose, remember the following:

- Before you start the activity, have a medical checkup and ask your health-care practitioner if the activity is suitable for you.
- Stop if you feel any pain and get advice before continuing.
- Always include warm-up and cool-down sessions (use the exercises from chapter 6) before you start and end any exercise session.
- Check that your teacher is fully qualified.
- Progress slowly.

WALKING

The benefits of walking are well known. For many people with arthritis, walking can be an ideal activity. It allows you to exercise the main muscles of the body. Doing a good warm-up before you go will ensure that your muscles are pliable and will make it easier and safer for you to get into a good walking rhythm. It is important to do some cool-down exercises at the end of the walk to help avoid fatigue and stiffness and return your muscles to their normal length.

There is very little risk of injury while walking as long as you take things slowly and do not do too much too soon. As you reach the end of the walk, it is sensible to slow the pace until you are strolling. Then do your cool-down and, if there is time when you get home, some deep relaxation.

Walking is less strenuous than other aerobic activities, but once you get into a good rhythm of brisk walking, you can burn as many calories in an hour as you can during a fast, 20-minute swim. It is also worth remembering that if you walk briskly for 30 minutes three to four times a week, you will improve your overall fitness and considerably reduce your risk of heart disease, obesity, diabetes, osteoporosis, stroke and certain cancers.

If you have done little or no exercise up until now or if your joints are painful, you will want to take things slowly. Walking for perhaps 10 minutes at a time to start with and building up to an hour over a period of weeks is a good idea. But even if you cannot walk for this length of time, the little you are able to do will still do you good.

You may also feel more comfortable if you alternate the speed at which you walk. Walk briskly for a while, then slowly for a bit and so on, until you feel comfortable walking briskly all the time.

Where you walk is up to you. You may prefer to use your car or bicycle to get to the nearest park or country path, but many people find it much easier to keep to a regular walking routine if they simply walk out of the front door and around the block.

You do not need any equipment for walking, apart from a pair of comfortable shoes—the best you can afford. They should give you good all-around support and have a cushioned sole. You may want to use extra inner soles as additional shock absorbers, particularly if you will be walking on hard pavement.

If you prefer to walk with others, check your local phone book or contact your local community college, YMCA or YWCA to find out if there are any walking groups in your area. You can also contact the American Volkssport Association, Suite 101, Phoenix Square, 1001 Pat Booker Rd., Universal City, TX 78148; 800-830-WALK.

SWIMMING AND
WATER EXERCISES

Water is a perfect medium for anyone with arthritis. The support it gives the body can allow you to do movements that are out of the question on dry land. Swimming is an excellent aerobic exercise that improves three major areas of fitness: mobility and flexibility, muscle endurance and aerobic fitness. Unlike other forms of exercise, it allows you to use all your muscles, and the more strokes you do, the greater the variety of movements you will put your muscles through. Because water cushions your body, the risk of injury is much reduced.

In addition to simply swimming lengths or widths, you may wish to try water exercises. When you exercise in water, you may feel as if you are not doing much, but in fact, you will be achieving a great deal.

You can try marching, first in place while holding on to the side of the pool, and then, if you feel confident, moving through the water. Wrist- and ankle-mobilizing exercises can also be done in water—in the bath as well as in the pool. If you wish to exercise in a pool, it is a good idea to do this with a friend who can offer encouragement and support. If you feel at all unsteady in the water, it is perfectly acceptable to wear armbands or rubber rings or to use plastic foam floats for support. But remember that these do not take the place of life jackets.

An alternative is to join a water exercise class. Many public swimming pools and fitness centers offer these, but before you sign up, make sure you have chosen a session that is right for you. Some combine swimming and aerobics and are quite demanding. The teacher should be properly trained in water exercise and should be able to advise you on what exercises to leave out if they are likely to exacerbate your condition.

If your arthritis is particularly bad, you may be able to have sessions in a **hydrotherapy** pool. Your physician should be able to arrange this. Often these sessions will be supervised by a physical therapist who will give you movements to do as well as help you into and out of the pool. The water in a hydrotherapy pool is a great deal warmer than that in the average public pool (usually more than 90°F), and this makes it easier to relax and really enjoy the feeling of being able to move with ease.

For many people, swimming is an ideal form of exercise. The only likely drawback is that unless the pool is very close, it may be difficult to get there three or four times a week. This is why people often combine swimming with other activities. Also, simply swimming laps can become very monotonous, so try using different strokes. Meditation techniques such as counting strokes, repeating a word or phrase or simply concentrating on the movements of your body will allow you to benefit mentally as well as physically.

CYCLING

This can be a relatively safe form of exercise for most people with arthritis. The non-weight-bearing pedaling movements do not jar the joints, although the constant repetition of movement involved may make cycling unsuitable for you if you have trouble with your hips or knees.

Cycling is enjoyable if the terrain is flat, if there is little or no traffic and if you are in the country, but if you live in a town or a hilly area, it may be less pleasurable and less suitable.

Again, you need to start slowly, choosing a short, flat route, then building up to something more demanding when you feel ready. Doing warm-up exercises before and cool-down exercises afterward is essential.

If you are thinking of buying a bike, remember that mountain bikes are good for off-road cycling but are heavy to carry. To pedal on the road, the standard touring bike suits most people, while a lightweight racing bike is wonderfully light to carry and makes hills a lot easier. Make sure the bike is the right size for your height. The most important measurement is the distance from the pedal to the seat, which should be a little longer than your pants inseam.

Cycling can also be a very sociable form of exercise. Many areas have cycling clubs, through which you can meet other enthusiasts. Check your local phone book or contact your local YMCA or YWCA to find out if there's a club in your area or contact the League of American Bicyclists, 190 W. Ostend St., Suite 120, Baltimore, MD 21230-3755; 410-539-3399.

YOGA

If you are looking for other ways to improve your flexibility and muscle strength, yoga is a good choice. In addition to helping your muscles, yoga can help you improve your breath control and learn to release tension. Yoga is completely noncompetitive. Each person does the different positions (*asanas*) to the best of her ability, never straining or overstretching.

Yoga sessions start with a period of relaxation and end with a meditation, which can be done sitting or lying down, depending on what feels most comfortable for you. Because the movements are performed so carefully and slowly, they are ideal for people with arthritis. They help improve strength and flexibility without straining the joints. But certain yoga positions, including The Plow, Neck and Hand Circles, and The Bow, are now recognized as being unsound for people with arthritis, so you should not do them. The meditation aspect of yoga can help you feel more at peace with yourself and the way you are.

Many of the *asanas* for beginners are simple, so you can practice them at home on your own, but starting with a class can give you a better idea of what yoga is all about. A good yoga teacher will be aware of current thinking and sensitive to the needs of his pupils. He will help you do as much as is comfortable and make sure you avoid any exercise that could hurt your joints such as those that involve kneeling. Check your local phone book or contact your local community college, YMCA or YWCA to find a class in your area.

ALEXANDER TECHNIQUE

This technique teaches you how to improve your posture. After a series of lessons, you will stand and move better and with more purpose. This could be especially useful if you suffer a lot of pain as a result of tension.

It is not possible to learn the Alexander technique from a book. You need to go to a trained teacher who will be able to show you how to establish the right coordination between your neck, head and back. You can then go home and gradually introduce these techniques into your daily life.

For more information about the Alexander technique, contact the North American Society of Teachers of the Alexander Technique, P.O. Box 517, Urbana, IL 61801; 800-473-0620.

FELDENKRAIS METHOD

Feldenkrais is similar to the Alexander technique in that it aims to reeducate you about the way you move.

Feldenkrais concentrates on the mastering of very small movements, and most exercises are done on the floor. The result is better posture. Feldenkrais can also reduce the amount of wear and tear on the joints—an important point if you have arthritis.

For more information about the Feldenkrais method, contact the Feldenkrais Guild, P.O. Box 489, Albany, OR 97321; 541-926-0981.

TAI CHI

Tai chi is an Asian martial arts discipline that centers on a series of slow, flowing rhythmic movements. It is very gentle, yet it can help you develop better balance and coordination as well as strengthen your muscles. Again, you need to go to a class to learn the movements, which you can then practice at home.

Tai chi encompasses a whole philosophy and approach to life. You do not have to adopt this philosophy in order to do the movements, but you may find that your attitudes and feelings gradually change. Check your local phone book or contact your local community college, YMCA or YWCA to find classes in your area.

WORKING OUT

Most fitness clubs offer a choice of circuit training, multi-gyms, weights and classes in step aerobics and other kinds of exercise. Most have the latest equipment, and you can tailor things to your needs and level of fitness. Some of the equipment may be quite useful for you. For instance, you may be able to have sessions on an exercise bike there rather than go to the expense of buying one of your own.

Before using any of the equipment, though, you should have a proper fitness assessment from a qualified staff member. You should be shown around and advised what equipment you should use and what you should avoid, depending on which of your joints are affected. An individual exercise program should be devised for you. You can then build on this program during the weeks and months that follow.

CHAPTER 9

Where to Find Out More

One of the most important things that you probably will have learned as a result of having arthritis is that you want to protect and comfort your inflamed and damaged joints as much as possible.

HOW YOU CAN HELP YOURSELF

There are several things that you can do to make life easier and relieve some of the stress on your joints:

- Unless rest is essential, try not to stay in one position for too long. When you are sitting, adjust your position frequently so that your joints do not become locked. When you are driving, stop at least every hour for a break.
- Learn how to use your back properly; always bend from the knees to pick things up.
- Make your life more efficient by cutting down on the number of tasks you do around the house. For instance, let dishes drip dry and use both hands when you pick things up.

There are many items available that can help make life easier, and it makes sense to look for them rather than struggle to cope without them. If you want to avoid bending, for example, look into one of the many types of reachers. These help you pick things up off the floor. If your grip is weak, try broad-handled cutlery, fat pens, handles for keys and plugs, tap turners and handles for turning knobs. Long-handled brushes and combs may also come in handy.

In the bathroom, you can overcome the problems associated with getting into and out of the tub by installing grab bars or by getting a bath insert. In the bedroom, make sure your bed is comfortable and look at the range of equipment that can make time spent in bed easier, such as pillow supports and book rests. For the garden, you can get long-handled, lightweight tools and special kneeling stools.

In short, there are very few areas of life that cannot be made easier for you with the right aid or piece of equipment. Most of these items can be bought, and some can be rented.

ABLEDATA, a national database sponsored by the National Institute on Disability and Rehabilitation Research, is a good source of information about assistive technology and rehabilitation equipment. The database contains information on more than 20,000 products from both domestic and international sources. For more information, contact ABLEDATA, 8455 Colesville Rd., Suite 935, Silver Spring, MD 20910; 800-227-0216, 301-588-9284.

You can also obtain useful catalogs from the following:

Accent on Living, P.O. Box 700, Bloomington, IL 61702; 800-787-8444

Aids for Arthritis, Inc., 3 Little Knoll Ct., Medford, NJ 08055; 609-654-6918

CLEO, Inc., Trent Building, South Buckhout St.,
   Irvington, NY 10533; 800-321-0595

Enrichments, P.O. Box 5050, Bolingbrook, IL 60440-
   5071; 800-323-5547

Maddak, Inc., 6 Industrial Rd., Pequannock, NJ 07440-
   1993; 800-443-4926

Patient's Personal Needs, Inc., 275 Centre St.,
   Holbrook, MA 02343; 800-289-4776

SUPPORT AND INFORMATION

A number of organizations can provide you with additional information about arthritis or help you find needed support or assistance. Below you will find contact information for several of these organizations, along with descriptions of the services they offer.

Ankylosing Spondylitis Association
P.O. Box 5872
Sherman Oaks, CA 91403
818-981-1616
800-777-8189
info@spondylitis.org
   Provides information on ankylosing spondylitis to consumers, health-care professionals and researchers. Maintains a library and conducts research.

Arthritis Foundation
1330 W. Peachtree St.
Atlanta, GA 30309
404-872-7100
800-283-7800
http://www.arthritis.org
   Provides a variety of services. Contact your local chapter, listed in the white pages of your phone book, to find out

exactly what services are available in your area. Services may include information about arthritis; referrals to doctors and clinics; help in finding local services; classes on self-care; exercise classes; clubs or support groups for people with arthritis; and discount drug services.

National Chronic Pain Outreach Association
P.O. Box 274
Millboro, VA 24460
540-997-5004

Provides information about chronic pain and its management. Operates an information clearinghouse for pain sufferers, family members and health-care professionals. A "Support Group Starter Kit" is available for the formation of local chronic-pain support groups.

National Institute of Arthritis and Musculoskeletal and
    Skin Diseases
NIH Information Clearinghouse
Box AMS
9000 Rockville Pike
Bethesda, MD 20892
301-495-4484

Collects, publishes and disseminates professional and public educational materials for people concerned with arthritis and related conditions. Offers a computerized research service.

COMPLEMENTARY THERAPIES

Some arthritis sufferers have found additional relief through complementary therapies. There are many such therapies from which to choose, but bear in mind that these treatments may not be covered by insurance. It is important to go to a qualified therapist. The best way to find one in your area is to approach an organization that represents the therapy. Here are a few you might like to try:

Acupuncture

American Association of Acupuncture and Oriental
 Medicine
433 Front St.
Catasauqua, PA 18032
610-433-2448
aaaom1@aol.com

National Commission for the Certification of
 Acupuncturists
1424 16th St., NW, Suite 501
Washington, DC 20036
202-232-1404

Chiropractic

American Chiropractic Association
1701 Clarendon Blvd.
Arlington, VA 22209
703-276-8800

International Chiropractors Association
1110 N. Glebe Rd., Suite 1000
Arlington, VA 22201
703-528-5000

Reflexology

International Institute of Reflexology
P.O. Box 12642
St. Petersburg, FL 33733-2642
813-343-4811
ftreflex@concentric.net

SUGGESTED READING

If you wish to learn still more about arthritis, you may find the following books helpful:

Arthritis Foundation Staff. *250 Ways for Making Life With Arthritis Easier.* Marietta, Ga.: Longstreet Press, 1997.

Arthritis Foundation Staff. *The Arthritis Foundation's Answers to All Your Questions.* Marietta, Ga.: Longstreet Press, 1997.

Cook, Allan, ed. *The Arthritis Sourcebook.* Detroit: Omnigraphics, Inc., 1997.

Irving, Ann F., Ann Kushner, Irving Kushner and the Arthritis Foundation Staff. *Understanding Arthritis.* New York: Macmillan, 1997.

Moyer, Ellen. *Arthritis: Questions You Have . . . Answers You Need.* Allentown, Pa.: People's Medical Society, 1997.

Pisetsky, David, M.D. *The Duke University Medical Center Book of Arthritis.* New York: Fawcett Columbine, 1991.

Sheon, Robert P., M.D., et al. *Coping With Arthritis.* New York: McGraw-Hill, 1987.

Sobel, Dava, and Arthur C. Klein. *Arthritis: What Works.* New York: St. Martin's, 1992.

Glossary

Acute: Beginning abruptly, then subsiding after a short period of time; sharp or severe.

Aerobic: Involving oxygen.

Ankylosing spondylitis: A type of arthritis that primarily affects the spine and sacroiliac joints. Tendons and ligaments may become inflamed where they attach to the bone. Advanced forms may result in the formation of bony bridges between vertebrae, causing the spine to become rigid.

Arthritis: Inflammation of joints; any of a number of rheumatic diseases involving joint inflammation.

Atrophy: Decrease in size of a normally developed organ or tissue; wasting.

Autoimmune disease: A disease caused by the action of the immune system against the body, occurring when the immune cells can't differentiate between the body's own material and foreign material.

Bone spur: A bony growth around a joint, seen in people with osteoarthritis.

Cartilage: A smooth, resilient tissue that covers the ends of bones so that they don't rub against each other.

Chronic: Developing slowly and persisting for a long time.

Connective tissue: Tissue that supports and connects internal organs, forms bones and the walls of blood vessels, attaches muscles to bone and replaces tissues of other types following injury.

Endorphins: Biochemicals that act on the nervous system to reduce pain and effect feelings of relaxation, pleasure and well-being.

Flare-up: A period during which symptoms worsen.

Gout: A form of arthritis caused by deposits of uric acid crystals in the joint. Gout usually strikes a single joint, often the big toe and often with sudden, severe pain.

Hydrotherapy: Any therapy that involves the use of water.

Inflammation: The body's protective response to an injury or infection. The classic signs—heat, redness, swelling and pain—are produced as a result of biochemicals secreted by the body's infection-fighting immune cells as they attempt to isolate and destroy any germs and to break down and remove damaged tissue.

Joint: A connection between bones.

Joint capsule: Tough, fibrous, fluid-filled tissue that completely surrounds a joint. Synovial cells lining the joint capsule secrete fluid to lubricate the joint.

Juvenile rheumatoid arthritis: A form of rheumatoid arthritis that develops in children.

Lactic acid: Organic acid present in body tissues, including muscles and blood.

Ligament: A thick, cordlike fiber that attaches bones to bones to keep them in correct alignment.

Lyme disease: A type of arthritis caused by bacteria transmitted by a tick.

Osteoarthritis: Degenerative arthritis, often caused by joint injuries or old age; the most common type of arthritis.

Osteoporosis: A condition in which bone mass and density decrease, making bones brittle and fragile.

Physical therapist: A health professional, trained and licensed in physical therapy, who helps physically disabled individuals regain functional movement, heal and adapt to their disabilities.

Range of motion: The range through which a joint can be extended and flexed.

Remission: Reduction or abatement of the symptoms of a disease.

Rheumatoid arthritis: A chronic disease in which inflammatory changes occur throughout the body's connective tissues.

Synovial fluid: Fluid secreted by the synovial membrane (the cells lining a joint capsule). It lubricates the joint and helps nourish the cartilage.

Synovial membrane: The cells lining the inside of the joint capsule that secrete lubricating fluid. In rheumatoid arthritis, the synovial membrane overgrows the joint capsule, invades the cartilage and begins to secrete biochemicals that can destroy a joint. Also called the *synovium*.

Systemic lupus erythematosus: Chronic, bodywide inflammatory condition that affects the joints, skin, blood, lungs, kidneys and cardiovascular and nervous systems.

Tendon: A strong band of tissue that connects muscle to bone.

Index

Note: Page numbers followed by asterisks indicate illustrations.

G

Gardening aids, 105
Gout, defined, 2, 111

H

Hydrotherapy, defined, 99, 111

I

Immune system, inflammation and, 1–2
Inflammation, defined, 1, 111
Information groups, 105–108

J

Joint
    arthritis effects, 1–2
    defined, 111
    osteoarthritis and, 3
Joint capsule, defined, 2, 112
Joints, guidelines to reduce stress, 104
Juvenile rheumatoid arthritis. *See* Rheumatoid arthritis,
    juvenile

L

Lactic acid, defined, 18, 112
Lifestyle, guidelines for easier, 104–105
Ligaments, defined, 2, 112
Lupus. *See* Systemic lupus erythematosus
Lyme disease, defined, 2, 112

M

Mobility. *See also* Warm-up exercises, mobilizers
    schedule, 29
Motor fitness, arthritis and, 10
Muscle endurance, arthritis and, 9–10
Muscle strength
    arthritis and, 9–10
    schedule, 29

O

Osteoarthritis
    causes, 3
    defined, 2, 3, 112
    effects, 3
    exercise and, 7